D0548572

Infant Psychiatry

DEVELOPMENTAL CLINICAL PSYCHOLOGY AND PSYCHIATRY SERIES

Series Editor: **Alan E. Kazdin**

In the Series:

Forthcoming:

Infant Psychiatry
An Introductory Textbook

Klaus Minde
Regina Minde

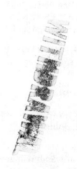

Volume 4.
Developmental Clinical Psychology and Psychiatry

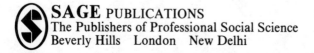

SAGE PUBLICATIONS
The Publishers of Professional Social Science
Beverly Hills   London   New Delhi

RJ
502.5
.M55
1986

Copyright © 1986 by Sage Publications, Inc.

All rights reserved. No part of this book may be reproduced or utilized in any form or by any means, electronic or mechanical, including photocopying, recording, or by any information storage and retrieval system, without permission in writing from the publisher.

For information address:

SAGE Publications, Inc.
275 South Beverly Drive
Beverly Hills, California 90212

SAGE Publications India Pvt. Ltd.
M-32 Market
Greater Kailash I
New Delhi 110 048 India

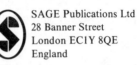

SAGE Publications Ltd
28 Banner Street
London EC1Y 8QE
England

Printed in the United States of America

Library of Congress Cataloging-in-Publication Data

Minde, Klaus, 1933-
  Infant psychiatry.

  (Developmental clinical psychology and psychiatry;
v. 4)
  Includes index.
  1. Infant psychiatry. I. Minde, Regina. II. Title.
III. Series. [DNLM: 1. Child Development. 2. Child
Psychiatry. 3. Infant. W1 DE997NC v. 4 / WS 350 M663i]
RJ502.5.M55 1985   618.92'89   85-14231
ISBN 0-8039-2519-0
ISBN 0-8039-2520-4 (pbk.)

FIRST PRINTING

CONTENTS

To Sally Provence,
who has shown us what an infant psychiatrist can be.

ACKNOWLEDGMENTS

Most of this book was written during a sabbatical leave in London and New Haven, which was financially assisted by the Laidlaw Foundation.

In addition to Sally Provence, whose continuing guidance and help has made this book what it is, we have profited from conversations and discussions with a large number of colleagues and friends. John Bowlby in London, William Kessen at Yale, and Hans Mohr in Kingston spent hours helping us to think historically about infancy and to translate developmental theories into a clinical assessment of an infant. Mel Lewis and Kyle Pruett helped us to get over the fear of writing such a book and showed us how to understand and treat a young child.

Maureen Dennis, Robert Harmon, Marian Sigman, and Paul Steinhauer critically read early versions of one or more chapters, and Peter Sutton and Jean Wittenberg, who share the senior author's day-to-day clinical work with infants, went through much of the manuscript on several occasions. Janet Britnell, who cheerfully typed the various versions of the book, never lost her courage and equanimity and must be given much credit for the final product.

Toronto

Klaus Minde
Regina Minde

SERIES EDITOR'S INTRODUCTION

Interest in child development and adjustment is by no means new. Yet only recently has the study of children benefitted from advances in both clinical and scientific research. Many reasons might explain the recent systematic attention to children including more pervasive advances in research in the social and biological sciences, the emergence of disciplines and subdisciplines that focus exclusively on childhood and adolescence, and greater appreciation of the impact of such influences as the family, peers, school, and many other factors on child adjustment. Apart from interest in the study of child development and adjustment for its own sake, the need to address clinical problems of adulthood naturally draws one to investigation of precursors in childhood and adolescence.

Within a relatively brief period, the study of childhood development, child psychopathology, and child mental health has evolved and proliferated considerably. In fact, several different professional journals, annual book series, and handbooks devoted entirely to the study of children and adolescents and their adjustment document the proliferation of work in the field. Although many different disciplines and specialty areas contribute to knowledge of childhood disorders, there is a paucity of resource material that presents information in an authoritative, systematic, and disseminable fashion. There is a need within the field to present latest developments and to represent different disciplines, multiple approaches to, and conceptual views of the topics of childhood adjustment and maladjustment.

The Developmental Clinical Psychology and Psychiatry Series is designed to serve uniquely several needs of the field. The series encompasses individual monographs prepared by experts in the fields of clinical child psychology, child psychiatry, child development, and related disciplines. The primary focus is on childhood psychopathology, which refers broadly here to the diagnosis, assessment, treatment, and prevention of problems of children and adolescents. The scope of the series is necessarily broad because of the working assumption, if not demonstrated fact, that understanding, identifying, and treating problems of youth regrettably cannot be resolved by narrow, single-discipline, and parochial conceptual views within a given discipline.

The task for individual contributors is to present the latest theory and research on various topics including specific types of dysfunction, diagnostic and treatment approaches, and special problem areas that affect adjustment. Core topics within child clinical work are addressed by the series. Authors are asked to bridge potential theory and research, research and clinical practice, and current status and future directions. The goals of the series and the tasks presented to individual contributors are demanding. We have been extremely fortunate in recruiting leaders in the fields who have been able to translate their recognized scholarship and expertise into highly readable works on contemporary topics.

The present book, devoted to the topic of infant psychiatry, has been prepared by Drs. Klaus Minde and Regina Minde. The book details the underpinnings of infant psychiatry in discussions of the nature of development including emotional, biological, and cognitive development. The significance of the topics becomes particularly clear in the clinical applications and research as illustrated in the detailed discussions of the psychiatric assessment of the infant, the measures and techniques that are available, and the problems that can emerge in their use. Major disorders are reviewed including pervasive developmental disorders, reactive attachment disorders, eating disorders, sleep disorders, and others. Treatment and recommendations for practitioners for diagnosing and managing dysfunctions that arise in infancy are elaborated as well. The book draws upon theory and research from multiple disciplines; the material is carefully integrated with case examples and concrete recommendations for clinical practice. The sum total of the individual chapters is an extremely authoritative and engaging text on the topic. We are very fortunate indeed to have Drs. Klaus Minde and Regina Minde as contributors to the series.

—Alan E. Kazdin, Ph.D.
Series Editor

1

HISTORICAL PERSPECTIVES

General child care attitudes and practices in North America today appear to be more inconsistent than they ever have been. On the one hand, knowledge about children has increased immensely over the last few decades and great importance is accorded today to the early years by many parents and professionals. On the other hand, the reported incidence of different forms of child abuse has also risen year by year. This is particularly disturbing to those among us who would like to believe that society can become more responsive and caring as our knowledge of the human condition increases. Despite our failure to prevent abuse, some modern historians of childhood find our record as a society an improvement over how children were treated in the past. Based on evidence of practices such as infanticide, early separation, and harsh physical handling, the history of childhood has, in fact, been called a "nightmare" from which we have begun to awaken only recently (de Mause, 1974).

In this chapter we will discuss some of the adverse experiences of infants in past centuries. We will also talk about some of the early parent advisers who have, for better or for worse, influenced society's understanding and handling of young children. Through this we hope to put into perspective our present outlook as clinicians on the developmental needs of young children and our attempts to satisfy these needs.

THE UNWANTED INFANT

Infanticide and Exposure

Called by Gibbon the "prevailing and stubborn vice of antiquity," the killing of infants, either directly by drowning or suffocating, or indirectly by exposure, was long considered an acceptable method to dispose of unwanted offspring among wealthy and poor parents alike (Langer, 1973/1974). As legend has it, Rome itself was founded by two exposed youngsters, Romulus and Remus, who had been rescued and raised by wolves. Infanticide was not even considered murder until the late fourth century in Europe, and was only sporadically punished prior to the sixteenth century. Tightening of the laws merely resulted in an increase in fatal "accidents" such as "overlaying"; that is, smothering in bed by parents or nurses, and in a surge of cases of abandonment (Hoffer & Hull, 1981; Hunt, 1970; Langer, 1973/1974; Trexler, 1973/1974). Such was the extent of the problem that some governments felt called upon to act on behalf of the victims. In the late eighteenth century both Austria and Prussia passed legislation making it illegal for children up to the ages of 5 and 2 respectively to share a bed with their parents (Langer, 1973/1974).

In many cities foundling homes were built to protect infants from death by exposure. Vincent de Paul, who became the patron saint of abandoned children, devoted his life to their rescue and care and established a foundling home in Paris in the seventeenth century (Henderson, 1953). Thomas Coram, a sea captain, worked for 17 years to have in 1741 a home opened in London, where the need was so great that in 1753 as many as 116 infants a day were offered for admission there (Caulfield, 1931); yet a century later it was still not uncommon to find dead babies in the streets of London (Langer, 1973/1974). The New York Foundling Hospital was not founded until 1869, prompted by the list of infanticides in each morning's paper (English, 1984).

The problem of unwanted offspring has been haunting us for thousands of years. Infanticide, whether tolerated or punished by society, has always been chosen as a way out by the unwilling parent when no other alternatives were available. Today, although methods of birth control such as the Pill are making it possible to avoid conception altogether, even they have failed to solve the problem. The much contended option of abortion, which for many is akin to infanticide, raises the question of how much things have changed fundamentally.

Early Separation

Another potentially destructive custom was the separation of infants from their mothers soon after birth, when they were sent out to be cared for by nurses for the first to third years of their lives. This was done not only by the well-to-do, but also by the less privileged, and was especially common in southern and western Europe in the seventeenth and eighteenth centuries (de Mause, 1974). A French statistic compiled by the chief of police in Paris in 1780 estimated that out of 21,000 babies born in that city every year, around 17,000 were sent out into the country to stay with professional wet-nurses, and between 2000 and 3000 babies of well-off parents were placed in suburban nursery homes. Another 700 were wet-nursed at home, while only about 700 were nursed by their mothers (Kessen, 1965; Robertson, 1974).

Wet-nurses were mothers whose own infants had died or been abandoned by them for economic reasons, thus enabling them to nurse the babies of more fortunate women instead. Judging from the thoughtful selection criteria we read about, for example, in Sainte Marthe's 1585 didactic poem "Paedotrophia" (Sainte Marthe, 1797), choosing a nurse was no light matter, and there is no reason to believe that most nurses were not decent, well-meaning people. But nurses have also been accused of smothering, neglecting, or abusing their charges (Hoffer & Hull, 1981; Hunt, 1970; Illick, 1974; Langer, 1973/1974). In cases where a nurse suckled another mother's baby in addition to her own, the unrelated child was often found to be neglected and to fail to grow satisfactorily (English, 1984).

The practice of hiring nurses, while accepted by society, was also resented by many. Since antiquity mothers were urged by poets, philosophers, and physicians to suckle their infants themselves. One argument was that nurses were less loving, that their affection was "spurious and constrained, for they love for hire" (Plutarch, quoted by Kessen, 1965). Another argument was that through the milk babies imbibed the morals of the nurse; since the natural mother was considered morally superior to a nurse, the baby was thought to benefit more from maternal nursing (McLaughlin, 1974). Rousseau went as far as predicting a renewal of the family and reform of morals when mothers would finally agree to nurse their own children. However, as we know, even he found it difficult to put this into practice. Not only did he separate his fictional child Emile from his mother, but he placed his own five children in an orphanage right after birth, against the protests of his common-law wife of many years (Rousseau, 1762/1979).

In general, evidence suggests that delegating the primary caretaking to a nurse was probably less widespread than has been suggested, nor was it necessarily a sign of the parents' indifference, if they resorted to this practice. While prevailing customs may have played a role, more often it may have been dictated by necessity, as in those cases where the mother had not enough milk or was too weak from frequent child-bearing to care for another newborn (Pollock, 1983). Before the days of the sterilized bottle, safe cow's milk, and infant formulas, many children would simply not have survived without the institution of the wet-nurse. Even with these life-saving conveniences the need for the nurse appears undiminished today, as witnessed by the extensive use by modern parents of daycare centers, nannies, and other types of child minders.

SHAPING THE INFANT IN THE IMAGE
AND FOR THE CONVENIENCE OF THE ADULT

Other child-rearing practices that have been frowned upon involve external constraints designed to influence the infant's physical growth, behavior, and development of character.

Swaddling

Infants have been swaddled since time immemorial. This was usually done with a long, two-inch wide band that kept the babies immobile, with their arms straight at their sides and their legs extended. A few extra turns around the head and, in some localities, a special stay behind both head and neck, helped to keep the head steady, so that only a small circle of the face was left exposed (Hunt, 1970; Marvick, 1974). Besides the major considerations of providing protection and warmth, swaddling was also considered an important way to ensure adultlike growth. Without this deliberate moulding, beginning at birth, children were long thought to risk retaining an immature shape and posture or even reverting to animallike locomotion. Pliny, in his *Natural History*, talked rather contemptuously about infants' need to wear "shackles," which together with their nakedness and wailing, proved to him that infants were even inferior to animals (Pliny, 1942). In the seventeenth century, the French physician Mauriceau still warned that if the child were not rigidly wrapped up in the prescribed way "so as to give his little body a straight figure, which is most decent and convenient for a man" he would go down "upon all fours as most other animals do" (Still, 1931).

Infants would remain in their swaddling clothes until they were about 3 or 4 months old, at which time their arms would be freed. After 8 or 9 months they would be released altogether and given sitting, standing, or running stools to assist them with their further motor development.

John Locke had some thoughts about the virtue of unrestrained movement, as we can see from his journals. He praised, for instance, the skill and ability of the Spartan nurses to bring up children without swaddling (October 3, 1678) and had a notion that the exercise of crawling may actually accelerate the attainment of walking. An entry on June 17, 1677, refers to infants on the Gold Coast, who, at 7 or 8 months, were left on the ground "so that you see them dragging themselves like kittens on four paws; this is also the reason why they walk earlier than European infants" (Dewhurst, 1963). But Locke never raised the issue in public. It remained for Rousseau, almost a century later, to proclaim freedom from swaddling as one of the principles of his natural way to raise children.

One aspect of swaddling not often mentioned is its calming effect on the organism. The authors of a modern study on this practice reported that infants who were swaddled tended to cry less, to sleep more, and to show a decrease in motor responsivity (Lipton, Steinschneider, & Richmond, 1965). In this respect, swaddling resembles another practice aimed at calming infants, the use of opium and alcohol.

Tranquilizing Infants

Opiates, for medicinal purposes, have been known to physicians for centuries, and opium-containing soothing syrups were prescribed for babies who had trouble falling asleep at least since Avicenna, around A.D. 1000 (Peiper, 1966). Such syrups were widely used, as the testimony of the English physician Curgeven before a parliamentary committee in 1871 shows. According to his report, 3000 children in Coventry alone were at that time treated with the infant tranquilizer Godfrey's Cordial, a concoction of opium, treacle, and sassafras, of which 10 gallons, or 12,000 doses, were sold weekly (Langer, 1973/1974). Alcohol was also given quite freely, either directly or indirectly through the milk of their nurses, so that gin was called the "real grand destroyer of infants," especially in eighteenth-century England (Caulfield, 1931).

Pediatricians condemned the custom of "dosing" or drugging babies (Still, 1931), and we assume that this kind of ignorance is for the most part a thing of the past. However, we wonder whether such treatment did not also have an adaptive function, similar to swaddling. Considering that an infant's continuing crying and fretting can be unsettling to the most understanding parents or caretakers and disturb some to the point of physical abuse, such attempts to restore peace may well have served at times to protect the child from worse treatment.

The Rod

The rod has historically been a symbol of parental authority. Most of us are familiar with it, and it is still a staple in many North American homes and classrooms. Yet the rod also used to have an undisputed place in the nursery. Even Locke, who argued so persuasively against its use, believed there were times when parents simply had to resort to physical punishment. As an example he relates the case of a "prudent and kind mother" of his acquaintance who was forced to whip her little daughter "at her first coming home from nurse [i.e., when the child had just been separated from an important caretaker] eight times successively the same morning before she could master her stubbornness and obtain compliance." He maintained that if the mother had left off sooner and stopped at the seventh whipping she would have "spoiled the child forever" (Locke, 1947). Whipping in such instances was obviously not practiced in anger, but thoughtfully, as a deliberate means of achieving compliance and teaching self-control, and sparing the adults and the children some trying experiences. Incidentally, the children of royalty were not treated with any more consideration than were those of commoners in this respect. We are told by Heroard, the physician appointed to look after young Louis XIII, that starting from his second birthday the Dauphin was beaten quite regularly, for example, for crying and for the refusal to eat or to show affection to his parents. Sometimes he had to expose his rear end for this purpose, so that the blows would fall on his bare behind (Hunt, 1970). But certainly whipping even young children has not gone out of fashion in our day. In a recent survey (Newson & Newson, 1976) it was found that 75% of British children had, by the age of 7, been hit with or threatened with implements ranging from wooden spoons and slippers to canes or belts.

ADULT INSENSITIVITY OR OVERINDULGENCE

Taken out of their historical and sociocultural context some of these practices appear to reflect a remarkable degree of insensitivity. On closer inspection, however, we invariably find some adaptive significance in them. Parents had to cope with two major problems, a lack of knowledge regarding family planning and high infant mortality. Children arrived unasked and they were so vulnerable to diseases and other hazards that about half of them died before they were 5 years old. No wonder if childhood, and particularly infancy, was thought of, by some, a less important phase of life, and that small children were "not worth much," in the words of a thirteenth-century poem, and "did not count," as Molière put it (both cited by Ariès, 1962), even if there were parents who would not have agreed. However, their precarious situation certainly should not lead us to believe that young children were not cherished. In fact, historical accounts, including the diaries of individual parents (Pollock, 1983), suggest that parental affection was the rule rather than the exception. Ariès quotes numerous writers who indeed resented the affection shown to small children since it reminded them of people's behavior toward little dogs or monkeys. Pliny, as we have seen, did not hide his contempt for infants, and since his books were widely read for centuries, his opinions were well known and possibly influential. Montaigne, the sixteenth-century humanist, admitted that he could not bear that "passion for caressing newborn children, which have neither mental activities nor recognizable bodily shape by which to make themselves lovable" (cited by Ariès, 1962). Likewise, Locke wrote his essay on education precisely because he felt parents were too indulgent with their little ones, showing them not just natural loving affection, which he thought "wisely ordained by nature," but often unwisely cherishing their faults as well (Locke, 1947). Two centuries later, the psychologist John Watson still felt that children needed to be protected from insensitive adults loving them "to death." As an example he related an experience he had with two boys aged 4 and 2 and their mother, grandmother, and nurse, when in the course of a two-hour ride, one of the children was kissed 32 times, and the other was almost equally "smothered with love" (Watson, 1928). Since there appear to be few female voices on the subject of the overindulgent parent, we assume that we are dealing here, as in so much of the literature on infants, with a male bias. Today the offending sentiment is regarded very highly as a biological and protective phenomenon—attachment. Pollock's study of parent-child relations between 1500 and 1900 (Pollock, 1983) confirms that on the whole parents were devoted to their offspring and clearly concerned about how best to raise them.

ADVISERS OF PARENTS

John Locke (1632-1704)

One of the most important messages of Locke's educational writings was that children were qualitatively different from adults and that these differences should be respected. While he still referred to the child as "incomplete" and to childishness as a "fault," he believed that "all their innocent folly, play and childish actions" were to be left perfectly free and unrestrained, because these were, as he put it, "faults of their age rather than of the children themselves," which should be "left to time and imitation and riper years to cure." Anticipating Rousseau, Locke wanted parents to inure their children to hardships and pain "that comes from the necessities of nature" and to withhold from them what they cry for, to prepare them for life's adversities. But he also admonished parents to let them play, to give them playthings, and even to encourage in them the "gainsome humour which is wisely adapted by nature to their age and temper." Since for Locke each infant was born a complex human being, he believed it was the parents' first task to observe him or her carefully in order to understand his or her individual "native propensities—predominant passions and prevailing inclinations" that the child had not yet learned to conceal. This would help them in their critical role as educators, "weeding out" their children's faults and "planting" good habits (Locke, 1947).

By raising the status of childhood in general and of the individual child in particular, Locke also emphasized the importance of the parent. His 1693 essay "Some Thoughts Concerning Education" was widely read and discussed on both sides of the Atlantic, and his influence was such that he has been called the Dr. Spock of the eighteenth century (Brant & Cullman, 1980).

Jean-Jacques Rousseau (1712-1778)

For Rousseau, as for Locke, children were born full of passions that had to be contained and channeled. They also agreed that infants came into this world infinitely malleable, which made child-rearing such a challenging task. But Rousseau did not share Locke's optimistic view that parents could be trusted to raise their children rationally. He saw them spoiling their children by either coddling or else neglecting them and by attempting to make them into adults before they were ready. Parents should understand that "nature wants that children are children before they become adults," that "childhood has its own way of seeing, thinking and feeling" and that it was therefore important to "treat them according to their age." Because of the special characteristics of childhood on the one hand and children's malleability on the other, Rousseau regarded this time as a critical period in human life that should not be wasted on formalized learning. The important thing was to exercise the child's "body, limbs, senses, and strength" as the tools of his or her later intelligence. Thus swaddling clothes were out; instead the infant was to crawl freely to allow his limbs to develop and stretch—"If you compare this child with one of the same age who has been kept carefully swaddled you will be surprised about the difference," parents were told. The child's mind, however, was to be left idle as long as possible. Instead, Rousseau sought to foster informal learning at every opportunity. As an example he mentioned the infant's stretching out his hand for a distant object, a gesture that Rousseau's contemporaries were likely to mistake as a desire to be in control, an order for the object to come or the caretaker to bring it to the child. In reality, Rousseau maintained, it meant that the infant's distance perception was not yet sufficiently developed to differentiate between far and near objects. Thus the caretaker should take the baby to the object in order to help him learn about distances (Rousseau, 1762/1979).

The issue of control loomed large in Rousseau's writings. A major principle of his child-rearing philosophy was that the child should never suspect the adult to be in control. For example, the guide or teacher in

Emile is advised to begin his task by observing first how nature exercises children continuously during their early years, hardening them by inflicting on them pain and illnesses. Accordingly, the power should always reside, or appear to reside, in the circumstances. Punishment, for instance, was never to be seen as an exercise of adult power, but as a natural consequence of the child's own actions. The caretaker had to become an expert behavioral engineer.

Rousseau knew that parents had a powerful influence on their children, and he attempted to minimize the potential harm parents could inflict by regulating their conduct. The reader is reminded here that Rousseau, like Locke, had little personal experience with young children. The two men to be introduced next, on the other hand, were professionals in the study of childhood.

Luther Emmett Holt (1855-1924)

Holt was a noted American pediatrician who opposed the use of opiates and the practice of swaddling and did much to improve the physical health of children. But he was also a proponent of strict and controlling parenting, advising parents never to give a child what it cried for but to prevent spoiling by letting it "cry out" to "break the crying habit." Moreover, he warned mothers not to play with babies under 6 months and "the less of it at any time the better," since this could cause all kinds of mental and physical problems. In keeping with this attitude, toilet training was to be started early, possibly in the second month of life (Holt, 1902).

Holt's opinions dominated nurseries for nearly half a century, as witnessed by the success of his book *The Care and Feeding of Children,* which was first published in 1894, went through 75 printings—the last in 1943—and was translated into Spanish, Russian, and Chinese.

John Broadus Watson (1878-1958)

Watson was a great admirer of Holt's principles and as concerned about the danger of spoiling children by unwise handling. He considered affectionate mothers their children's worst enemies, calling "mother love" a "dangerous instrument" to blame for everything from an unhappy infancy to an unhappy marriage. Mothers were therefore told by Watson to hold back their feelings for their children, as by kissing them, picking them up, and rocking them, they were "slowly building up a human being totally unable to cope with the world it must later live in." If mothers were too tenderhearted, they could watch their little ones through a periscope or a peephole from an adjacent room. In order to protect young children from affection, Watson even considered raising them in a community of homes with well-trained nurses who could circulate so that the babies were fed and bathed each week by a different nurse and would not become attached to any one of them (Watson, 1928).

While obviously concerned about the rights of the small child and the duties of parents, these "experts" were oddly out of tune with either, although to a degree they may have helped advance the case of infancy as a state of its own, worth thinking and writing about. They helped to do away with customs such as swaddling that had restricted the infant's movements and growth. On the other hand, they told mothers to mistrust their natural feelings toward their children and become behavioral engineers; that is, ever better at controlling them. This functional approach to child-rearing influenced generations of middle-class parents more or less until the advent of those supporters of responsive mothering, Dr. Spock (1946) and Selma Fraiberg (1959).

ADVOCATES OF MOTHERS

Of course, the importance of responsive mothering had been "scientifically" established centuries ago. As we learn from Salimbene, Frederick II, Emperor of the Holy Roman Empire, allegedly induced a sample of foster mothers and nurses not to talk to the infants they cared for so that he might find out what language they would naturally produce: Hebrew, Greek, Latin, Arabic, or the language of their natural parents. He received no answer to his question, because the children all died "for they could not live without the petting and joyful faces and loving words of their foster mothers" (Ross & McLaughlin, 1949).

The most eloquent advocate of mothers as the most important natural allies of their infants, even when untrained, was the Swiss educator Johann Heinrich Pestalozzi (1746-1827). He was at first excited about Rousseau's ideas, named his first son, born in 1770,

Jean-Jacques, and tried to raise him after the model of Emile, but he later dissociated himself from Rousseau. For Pestalozzi maternal love was the first agent in education. He praised the mother for opening the world for her infant by following only her instincts. "She makes him ready to use his senses and prepares for the early development of his attention and power of observation" (Pestalozzi, 1900). According to his own account he took the inspiration from an unnamed woman in Appenzell who hung a large colorful paper bird over her baby's cradle, which the 2- to 3-week-old infant greeted with outstretched hands and feet. Here, he said, the mother showed clearly the point at which the art of education should begin to bring the objects of nature firmly to the child's clear consciousness. If the mother could be, out of herself, so sensitive to her infant's competencies, how much better would she be if properly trained? Pestalozzi based on his observation a whole system of guidelines for education "at the knee," for teaching and stimulating infants "even before they are able to utter a single sound," firmly anchored in the mother-child dyad. These guidelines were published in a series of letters in 1801 (Pestalozzi, 1900) and established him as one of the forefathers of today's infant training programs, along with Froebel and Montessori.

THE CHILD AS AN OBJECT OF STUDY

Another group of people whose work has influenced our present understanding and treatment of young children were the early baby biographers, foremost among them Charles Darwin (1809-1882). His insights into the history of the human species suggested to him the scientific value of studying the development of the child as one way to learn more about the evolution of man. He himself led the way by carefully observing and recording the day-to-day behavior of his first child, William Erasmus, called Doddy, in 1841-1842. An account of this diary, which showed Darwin as a kind and patient father as well as an astute observer, was later published in the journal *Mind* in 1877. Here Darwin imparts to the reader his sense of wonder and respect for the competency of the infant. He was especially interested in his son's affective development and intrigued by his precocious ability to interpret—as early as 5 months—the "meaning and feelings" of his caretakers from the expressions on their faces (Darwin, 1877).

Baby watching has, of course, become a most fruitful and popular pastime among students of development since Darwin's time, and has continued to broaden our understanding of infancy, from Piaget's and Gesell's germinal observations of child behavior in the 1920s and 1930s to the most recent ethological observations of parents and infants in the premature nursery.

CONCLUSION

We have no way of knowing how reliable the historical sources on this subject are, but there is no doubt that many infants have suffered in the past through adult ignorance and insensitivity. At the same time, present-day statistics and clinical accounts of abuse and abandonment remind us that for many children life remains a nightmare, and, moreover, that the abusing parent of today is raising the abusing parent of tomorrow (Bowlby, 1984). On a more general level, we have to concede that the status of the infant in our society has undergone changes. He has evolved from an incomplete, if likable, being of little consequence to one who has become the focus of scientific inquiry and emerged as much more clever and adaptable than had ever been suspected. This has come about partly because of the advocacy of some thoughtful physicians and educators in the past and partly because medical advances have strengthened the infant's formerly precarious hold on life.

As a society we like to see ourselves today as more sophisticated, caring, and in tune with infants, as we have learned more about them and, by means of birth control, increased the likelihood that more children born are wanted. Still, we cannot prevent some of them from becoming targets of abuse, and we have been unable to bridge the gap between those who see and accept babies from within their developmental perspective and those who approach them as an extension of our adult society, in need of training and change. Hence their status in our society remains ambiguous.

Finally, this brief historical overview shows that some of our contemporary concepts of infancy are not as novel as we may have thought, and that, as Kessen pointed out, the history of child study is a "history of rediscovery" (Kessen, 1965).

2

GENERAL PRINCIPLES OF NORMAL INFANT DEVELOPMENT

Infant psychiatry as a medical specialty has both a clinical and educational mandate. On the one hand its practitioners assess and treat those young children who have difficulties in meeting the normal expectations of their families and society at large. In addition, however, mental health professionals also assemble knowledge about children's emotional, cognitive, and social needs and make it available to those who assist children in their growth and development.

In the following chapters we describe a number of psychiatric syndromes and abnormal behavioral manifestations occurring in children under age 3. We will show how particular environmental and constitutional forces influence or possibly even cause some of these symptoms and point out possible ways to modify their deleterious consequences. Yet common to all these investigative, diagnostic, and treatment efforts must be the awareness that disturbed infants show deviations in some aspects of their emotional, social, or cognitive development.

Since it follows that it is impossible to understand the psychological problems of infants without an adequate appreciation of normal developmental events and the role families have in this process, we will devote this chapter to giving an overview of some aspects of development and family functioning in young children. We will first discuss some general developmental principles that will allow us to see the features common to various theories of human development. Then the effects of particular theoretical developmental principles on the understanding of specific aspects of child development during the first three years will be illustrated. The physical development of children as well as some aspects of their cognitive growth will not be discussed. Our primary emphasis on understanding clinical deviance in young children, and the book's space limitations, made these selections necessary.

GENERAL DEVELOPMENTAL PRINCIPLES

As pointed out in Chapter 1, there had been little interest in an objective examination of the development of children until the last century. Only when society provided educational experiences for the majority of children did psychologists and pediatricians look at children's behavior and development because education eroded the previously rigid intergenerational social structure and offered individuals the possibility of choosing an occupation other than that of their parents. Hence, it suddenly had become important to predict who could make use of these new opportunities and to learn more about those who could not.

The traditional concept of development since Darwin had the predeterministic notion that "ontogeny recapitulates phylogeny" (that is, the development of the individual repeats that of the species). This notion was based on the understanding that the human embryo in the course of intrauterine development passes through each stage of the evolutionary process, from the single cell via the fish or reptile stage to its final mammalian form. Psychologically, this implied that human and animal behavior was closely related and that children were endowed with the sins and failures of their phylogenic ancestors.

Various scientific advances during the later part of the last century called the predeterministic position of development into question. Scientists and clinicians recognized that the physical or psychological characteristics an individual inherits (that is, his or her genotype) may not be identical with the psychological or physical characteristics an individual shows (that is, his or her phenotype), but that the phenotype reflected the genetic base after its modification by the environment.

However significant questions remained about how development, in fact, proceeded. One group of investigators (Baer, 1970) felt that changes in the behavior or abilities of young children occurred steadily and varied little over time. This implied that learning as well as development were smooth and even processes that would vary only in response to the input the environment provided for the organism. On the other hand, a considerable group of clinicians and theorists stressed, based on much clinical and research evidence, that development proceeds in clearly defined stages (Piaget, 1952; A. Freud, 1946). This stage, or "epigenetic," concept of development was based on the observation that certain groups of behaviors routinely appear together. For example, children begin to show marked stranger anxiety (a milestone in their emotional development) usually around the time they can recognize the differences between strange and familiar faces (a cognitive developmental achievement). While there is still much debate whether this cognitive skill must first be established to allow the emotional reaction to strangers to occur or whether the reverse is true, the epigenetic theory implies that both of these new behaviors are followed by other specific functions. In our example, the differential recognition between strange and familiar faces will be followed by the child's ability to recall his or her mother's face even when she is not physically present. This then allows children to explore areas of their environment without being anxious regardless of their mothers' presence or absence. This in turn facilitates new learning and competence. Epigenetic theories therefore suggest that new behaviors occur only if their more elementary precursors have been mastered and have strong biological underpinnings.

Another question deriving from the stage or epigenetic model concerns the extent to which each stage is indeed a necessary precursor for the following stage or to what degree developmental steps will occur independently from each other—that is, are discontinuous. While for some investigators "the cumulation of early life experiences, beginning in infancy, is critical for and determinative of later development and behavior" (Lipsitt, 1983, p. 63), others observe that "many instances of developmental change can be characterized by replacement of an old structure by a new one, with little or no connection between the two hypothetical structures" (Kagan, 1981, p. 68). Those conflicting views reflect some of the most lively controversies besetting present-day psychology. While a detailed discussion of these issues is beyond the scope of this volume, we will at least give a brief sketch here. Rutter, in a recent chapter on the continuities and discontinuities in socioemotional development (Rutter, 1984), describes some of the pitfalls in the usage of the term "developmental continuity" by various scientists. He points out that the notion of continuity can mean the unchanging persistence of a quality, such as the ability to form a bond to another person, which does not usually disappear once it has been acquired. It can also imply, however, a regularity in the pattern of development as documented by the fact that monozygotic twins show a greater concordance than dizygotic twins in their intellectual development over time (Wilson, 1977).

Other forms of continuity have been labeled "ipsative stability." This term refers to the stability within an individual in respect to various personality variables such as temperament (Emmerich, 1968). It also refers to the notion that individuals, at least after they have achieved a certain degree of biological and cognitive competence, seek their own environment and hence tend to maintain stability.

Finally, there is the supposed continuity in a particular internal structure of an individual. For example, Bowlby (1969, 1980) has suggested that close personal relationships developed early in life can serve as a protective function throughout life. Bowlby does not say that these relationships are identical when a person is 2 or 60 years old or that their quality is related across various ages. However, he does suggest that the relationships a person makes at any age involve the same internal structures and represent a continuity of the self.

While more details and practical examples of these issues will be given in later sections of this chapter, we must make brief reference to some data that are often used to document the discontinuity of development. The most convincing studies in this area are those that show that intelligence as measured during the first 18 months of life has virtually no correlation with later intellectual ability (McCall, 1981). Likewise, early behavioral patterns of sleeping irregularity, the amount of crying, or the facility of feeding do not usually continue beyond infancy, and problems in these areas do not predict other difficulties at later times. While their causes are not fully understood, various authors have stated that these discontinuities are related to biologically determined cognitive or emotional reorganizations or behavioral transformations (McCall, 1981). This concept implies that at specific times in a person's life there occurs a total reorganization of his or her behavior. For example, a 2- to 3-month-old infant suddenly shows a social smile; that is, he or she responds to a familiar figure by smiling. A baby at that time also usually consolidates his or her wake-sleep cycle and has established a stable pattern to fit habituation to visual and auditory stimuli. This means that from an organism dominated to a significant degree by reflex behaviors, the baby has suddenly become a powerful contributor to social interactions with his or her environment. Most important, however, is the finding that an infant who is poorly regulated and organized at 6 weeks does not have less chance of developing adequate social behaviors at 3 months than has a baby who was easy and regular during his or her early weeks.

While the examples we gave for the discontinuity of development dealt with intelligence and facets of the infant's cognitive, biological, and social nature, later periods of behavioral reorganization can also involve areas of emotional importance. For example, there is now good evidence that repeated hospitalizations of children between the ages of 6 months and 5 years have psychologically detrimental effects, at least into late adolescence (Quinton & Rutter, 1976). Yet children under the age of 6 months and those older than 5 years seem not to be adversely affected. While the reason for these differences is not known, it seems possible that the different maturation of various cognitive and emotional functions will allow the organism to approach the world around it in qualitatively very different ways at specific developmental periods.

There are two more basic principles that differentiate developmental theories: the degree of activity assigned to the infant within his or her interactional system and whether there is an optimal endpoint to development.

Traditionally, the mother or parent was seen as the main determinant of a child's behavior (Freud, 1965; Sears, Maccoby, & Levin, 1957) although biologically oriented scientists such as Gesell and Amatruda (1964) emphasized the almost automatic unfolding of new behaviors. Common to both positions is the relative passivity of the infant. Thus the baby was shaped either by his or her caretaker or by the indigenous buddings of new developmental competencies. However, more recent work has stressed the degree to which children shape their own environment either through their sex or state of alertness (Moss, 1967), temperament (Thomas, Chess, Birch, Herzog, & Kern, 1963), or basic interactional repertoire (Brazelton, Yogman, Als, & Tronick, 1979).

The question of whether there is an optimal endpoint to development is rarely addressed directly in developmental theories. However, in general we find that more traditional developmentalists perceive adulthood or the achievement of formal operational thinking as an endpoint of development (Gesell & Amatruda, 1964) while learning theorists and other recent writers see life as an ongoing unfolding of newer developmental problems and solutions (Baltes, Reese, & Lipsitt, 1980; Erikson, 1959; Sameroff & Chandler, 1975).

DEVELOPMENTAL THEORIES

There have been many theories of human development, well summarized by Hall and Lindzey (1970). Among these, the theories derived from psychoanalytic thinking, the organismic concepts of Werner (1948), and general behaviorism have had such a powerful influence on our understanding of the behavior of young children that a more detailed discussion of them seems in order.

The Psychoanalytic Approach

Psychoanalytic theory of child development is but one part of the much larger theoretical structure of psychoanalysis. S. Freud, the founder of psychoanalysis, saw human behavior as an expression of instincts or drives, innate derivatives of our species' striving for self-preservation (Freud, 1953). These drives, which were given different names at different stages of Freud's own thinking, were seen to represent an individual's needs, wishes, or desires for pleasure and survival. As an individual's pleasures are often in direct opposition to the social organization of others, conflicts are inevitable. Such conflicts usually lead either to the blockage (repression) or modification (sublimation) of instincts to fit socially acceptable norms. From a developmental point of view, Freud's theory implies that conflict is an essential part of development and the aim to solve innate conflicts the main motor of developmental progression and learning. Freud's later writings suggest (Freud, 1952) that the inherently biological part of man is represented by the hypothetical mental structure of the "id." This structure aims at a rapid and complete discharge of drive energy, does not follow laws of logic, and is therefore described as using "primary processes."

The second principle of psychoanalysis is the assertion that much of the compromising between the instincts and society occurs outside our awareness in the unconscious. This is because we all develop powerful defensive mechanisms such as denial, projections, or reaction formations to deal with the innate conflicts between our id drives and society's laws and regulations and to prevent the conflicts from becoming fully conscious. According to Freud these defensive maneuvers are generated by the "ego" and the "superego." The ego is a structure that is said to represent external reality within the psyche. In that sense it must find ways to prevent the blatant expression of id impulses yet also allow some discharge of tension. It regulates the expression of the id and also tests the reality of a person's environment. Later in life, the ego is supported by the superego, which is essentially the hypothetical intrapsychic structure that represents learned cultural standards. While the ego signals a conflict between instinctual desires and society's demands by making a person anxious, the superego, when in conflict, causes feelings of guilt and in this way inhibits instinctual expression.

Finally, there are those principles of psychoanalysis most important for early child development, namely the postulated series of different instinctual forces that become sequentially active possibly as a result of biological maturation. If they were either insufficiently satisfied or received too much gratification, the individual would continue to desire childhood gratifications in adult life, and especially following stressful experiences, exhibit "regressive behaviors." According to Freud, these behaviors mirror the instinctual period on which the child is "fixated"; that is, the period during which his or her needs had been least adequately satisfied. The instinctual oral, anal, and phallic stages were thought to be related to specific developmental periods.

The last stage of development occurring in young children, the phallic stage, is described as characterized by the child's fascination with his or her external genitalia and the general categorization of his or her environment into old and young people, mothers, grandmothers, boys and girls, and the like. Freud believed that during the phallic stage children, for reasons specified later in this chapter, are especially drawn to the parents of the opposite sex (Oedipus complex) and that fixations to this phase would show themselves later in unsatisfactory heterosexual relationships.

While Freud's early categorization of developmental stages has been extensively modified and expanded by later psychoanalytic workers such as E. Erikson (1963), A. Freud, (1965) and M. Mahler (1968), all these theorists follow the epigenetic developmental model and suggest that a child has to pass from stage A to stage B before he or she can reach stage C. They also share the concepts of regression and fixation points, talk about the same defense systems, and agree that symptoms displayed by a child will have a psychological meaning that can only be understood from his or her life history and previous development.

Since the advent of ego psychology initiated in particular by the writings of Hartmann (1958), biological characteristics have also been represented in concepts of an "ego constitution." These are inborn somatic apparatuses such as motility, intelligence, memory, speech, and a general organizing function that underlie specific ego functions.

The Organismic Approach

The organismic approach to development had its historical roots in work by early twentieth-century biologists who experimented with transplanting tissues in certain animal embryos from one anatomical location to another. These researchers found that the tissues (for example, an arm) when grafted before the organism had reached a particular age would take on the characteristics of the tissue area where they were placed (for example, a leg). However, after a specific age, the transplanted arm tissue would retain its original structure. This suggested that there existed a "developmental organizer" the effects of which could not be altered by later environmental changes. Such an organizing principle has also been thought to be present in the area of psychological development (Werner, 1948). For example, Werner stressed that the development of any function proceeded from a relatively global to a differentiated functional state and that these differentiated parts were then organized in a hierarchical system.

However, recent work has shown that even newborn infants exhibit far more highly organized specific behaviors than had previously been reported. These behaviors primarily reflect the internal state of the infant and among others consist of sucking and crying rhythms or cycles in sleep-wakefulness (Anders & Weinstein, 1972; Prechtl, 1974; Wolff, 1966, 1969).

Many rhythmic and other simple as well as complex motor behaviors have also been regularly observed in fetuses as soon as 10 weeks after conception. This places such movements ten weeks earlier than had been thought possible only very recently (Prechtl, 1985).

The concept of an organizing principle has recently been extended by Sameroff and Chandler (1975) in an attempt to throw new light on the interactions between an organism and its environment. Thus Sameroff and his colleagues believe that most behaviors in children are guided by a "self-righting principle," which will be triggered into action in an attempt to realign the behavior in question if things move too far away from the median. This realignment can come both from within the child (for instance, a baby may suddenly fall asleep when he or she gets overstimulated) or from the environment (for example, fathers of twins are more significantly involved in the day-to-day care of their infants than are fathers of singletons as mothers simply cannot cope well enough alone; Marton, Minde, & Dawson, 1981). This means that one can see "organizers" as both biological and cultural social phenomena, the latter being transmitted through general cultural or family channels.

The organismic approach does not concern itself directly with the question of the epigenesis of behavior although Wolff (1966) and Prechtl (1985) certainly conceptualize that a child develops according to preset stages. On the other hand, theorists subscribing to an organismic model would see the child as playing a very active part in the process of this development. They would also conceptualize development to go on all through life and allow novel tasks and experiences to lead to behaviors that could not necessarily be predicted from earlier interactions or life experiences.

The Behavioral Approach

While the previously discussed developmental theories are anchored in the biological maturation of the human organism, behaviorists claim that both the behavioral and cognitive repertoires of an individual can best be accounted for by his or her past experiences. Beginning with Locke's and Rousseau's educational concepts through Watson's (1924) and Skinner's (1953) understanding of how certain contingency patterns can shape behavior, and most recently in Kagan's (1982) review on the development of children who had experienced early deprivation, there has been the contention that the present behavior of an individual is a reflection of his or her previous interactions with his or her environment. The philosophical foundations of this approach to development have come from many sources, ranging from politicians who believed in freeing humanity from the shackles of slavery or other social bondage, to educators who tried to free people from ignorance. Yet varying theories have undergone significant changes over the years. For example, early behaviorists had little understanding of the limitations neuronal maturation placed on a child's ability to learn both motor and cognitive tasks. They also thought that learning was primarily mediated through observable interactions and largely ignored such powerful structures as the need for human contact or attachment, which motivate and hence influence so much of our everyday learning and behavior. However, recent work by Bowlby on the attachment of children and adults (1969, 1973, 1980) and its experimental validation by Sroufe (1979) and many others have clearly influenced the thinking of modern behaviorists. For example, they now talk about "internal mediators" and their power to modify external experiences.

A good example of the complexity of current learning theory is the work of Bandura (1977). However, in our opinion the behavioral or learning theories, in contrast to psychoanalytic theory, have not been able to account for the immense variety and richness of human behavior. They have, however, through their emphasis on testing and modification of hypotheses, contributed immeasurably to the clarification of many issues pertinent to learning and development. Proponents of learning theories have also believed in the ever-continuing process of development since growth and new learning can obviously take place until death. Finally, they clearly acknowledge the contribution children make to their own developmental fate although much emphasis is given to the facilitating environment needed for healthy growth and development.

CURRENT STATE OF KNOWLEDGE

This brief review of three developmental concepts should make clear that child development can be viewed in various ways. Yet despite this diversity, there is a general agreement on some points.

First, scientists recognize today that no single concept of development can do justice to all the phenomena we see in developing children. The question of to what extent development is continuous or discontinuous cannot be answered globally. Thus, as Rutter (1984) has pointed out, we have realized that continuity is not the same as constancy or stability and that we may be better served if we looked for meaningful links over the course of development. We also know that some functions, such as cell growth, occur continuously although even in this area we can see spurts of growth occurring at specific times. Other functions, such as a child's particular way of thinking or his or her use of language, proceed in stages and seem to follow a logical sequence, linking previous with later developmental tasks and abilities. For example, the ability to move about can be used for exploration and learning much more effectively if the child has incorporated an image of his or her mother without her being physically present.

In support of the epigenetic developmental theory is the finding that there is a lower limit for the appearance of many developmental phenomena that is determined primarily by the maturation of the central nervous system responsible for the task in question. For example, no amount of stimulation will make a child walk, run, or talk by the age of 5 months. However, verbal and physical stimulation does play an important part in preparing the ground for the acquisition of these skills as without this they will emerge significantly later (Provence & Lipton, 1962).

In addition to these inherently meaningful links in a child's development, there are other events that provide no such obvious connections but seem to be based on a complete reorganization of an organism (Hinde, 1982). The social smile and its accompanying new attachment behavior at age 6 weeks and the increase in depressive feelings at puberty are examples here. They may be caused by genetically determined maturational changes (smiling) or by an increase in hormonal activity at puberty (depression). Yet both events present a discontinuity from previous behaviors although they are of course influenced by the physical status of the organism and a specific psychosocial environment.

Second, most social scientists acknowledge that children are important shapers of their environments. Children do not merely react to their environment, the environment reacts to them as well. Findings of this nature have led to an increasing number of infant studies that include the parents and look at both sides of the interactional system simultaneously to learn how the participants adapt to each other (Sander, 1970; Stern, 1974). Such studies have also taught us that parental feelings, attitudes, and responses will be influenced by the degree to which an infant meets the parents' preexisting needs and tolerance. The more their needs are satisfied, the easier parents will find it to accept and value their child and the greater will be their ability to provide him or her with the environment he or she needs for optimal growth.

A further consequence of both the principles of maturation and reorganization within the social context is the possibility that a specific developmental task can be reached by different routes. The behavioral reorganization that occurs at different ages, for example, may cause early less adaptive behaviors of the child or his or her caretakers to become irrelevant for later adaptation. This in turn can help new behavioral patterns to work toward a previously unachieved goal. For example, a mother who has been uncomfortable for whatever reason in providing close physical contact to her little daughter during the first 6 months of her life and hence has failed to establish the prerequisites for a secure attachment may be able to give the child her undivided supportive attention when she begins to explore the world around her during the second part of the first year. This will permit the child to feel sufficiently confident about herself to go on with her development without any significant conflict. Likewise, children who are congenitally blind or who are born without limbs may not encounter the sensory motor experiences normally associated with healthy development. Yet studies by Fraiberg (1977) and Decarie (1969) have shown that most of these children in the end develop good intelligence and self-awareness in early childhood.

Another common principle is that development is not a phenomenon that affects only one sphere of life, such as intelligence or physical growth, but the sum total of forces that embrace changes in biological, cognitive, emotional, and social behavior. While researchers have claimed previously that specific advancements in cognitive development are prerequisites for new advances in other areas, such as the emotional development of a child, the present consensus is that all areas of development constantly interact and influence their mutual progression (Belsky, 1981). Therefore, all areas of development should be examined when assessing a child for a possible deviation in only one area of development.

3

PATTERNS OF NORMAL INFANT DEVELOPMENT

The preceding chapter has given a general overview of important developmental principles as seen by various theorists and pointed out areas of agreement and disagreement between them. It also stressed the recent focus on the interactional aspects of development and the need to see this process as a reflection of the interplay between all the child's developmental parameters and his or her environment. We will now examine the expected manifestations of a child's biological, social, cognitive, and emotional development more systematically and see how they interact and influence the child's day-to-day behavior.

BASIC DEVELOPMENTAL PARAMETERS

Motor and Cognitive Development

An infant's motor and cognitive development, like other behavioral repertoires, is characterized by specific discontinuities at around 2, 9, and 18 months. A discussion of a child's development during the first three years is therefore best subdivided into the four periods suggested by these shifts.

Birth to 2 months. The newborn infant shows many behaviors that have been described as "endogenous" both in origin and aim. Thus much of the infant's activity is thought to be stimulated by changes that originate within him or her, giving the impression that he or she is relatively isolated from outside stimuli. These internal events are called "states" and refer to certain patterns of physiological variables or behaviors that repeat themselves and are stable within themselves (for example, crying, fussing, quiet alertness, drowsiness, active or quiet sleep; Prechtl, Akiyama, Zinkin, & Kerr Grant, 1968). Peter Wolff, who was one of the first scientific baby watchers, soon recognized that the state the newborn is in is intimately linked to his ability to process information and respond to his environment (Wolff, 1966). Thus a baby who cries or fusses will be much less likely to take in outside events than will an infant who is quietly alert. More important, the association between states and interactive potential has opened the door to studies that have tried to modify the length of certain stages such as wakefulness (Wolff, 1966) so as to allow the infant to gain more external input. Furthermore, they have stimulated a good deal of work and questions such as: How do infants move from state to state? Are there individual differences? Can infants calm themselves without outside help (Brazelton & Als, 1979)? If not, how can we best help them (Korner & Thoman, 1972)? While a detailed discussion of these studies would go beyond the scope of this chapter, one can say, as Emde and Robinson (1979) have put it, that newborns are active and seek to optimize exposure to informative aspects of their visual world (p. 86). In other words, the young organism is programmed not so much to shut out stimulation but to seek it in areas that are important for its neuronal and interpersonal growth. Hartmann (1958) referred to this as the human infant's being born "preadapted" to an average expectable environment.

The motor behavior of the infant during this period outwardly appears to support the notion of the inward-directed organism. Newborn infants sleep 85% of the time (Anders, 1974), have virtually no control over their posture, and will not reach or grasp anything. They actively display a number of reflexes (for example, the Moro, automatic walking, and tonic/neck reflex). However, these reflexes normally disappear during the early months of life.

2 to 9 months. At around 8 to 10 weeks babies accomplish a number of motor feats that reflect an important qualitative change in their biological development, namely the ability to shift from endogenous to exogenous control. Infants can now control their heads and in that sense determine when to look at the world. They also begin to bring their hands together and engage them in playful mutual fingering by 16 weeks. They can retain objects in their hands, albeit briefly, and a bit later are beginning to reach out for both objects and people. All these functions are perfected during the ensuing six to eight months, which make them much more active initiators of and responders to outside events. Other patterns also change. For example, there are very marked changes in sleep states, with a doubling of quiet sleep and a corresponding decrease of REM sleep at 8 to 10 weeks of age (Emde & Metcalf, 1970). Infants learn to sleep through the night to a significant degree (Kligman, Smyrl, & Emde, 1975; Parmelee, 1974) because of the shift from irregular and almost random distribution of waking and sleeping stages to a more diurnal mode of nighttime sleep. Parallel to these changes we find that at this time infants learn to organize or console themselves far more easily than before by sucking their thumb or engaging in other self-soothing behaviors. Similarly, infants can be habituated readily from this time onward, which means that environmental phenomena are potentially far more powerful in modifying the expectations and behavior of an infant after 8 weeks of life (Lipsitt, 1983).

Finally, infants at about 2 months will be attracted to stimuli that fit into a familiar schema, that is, patterns they have seen before (Fantz & Nevis, 1967). Stimuli that are either too familiar or too discrepant from that scheme will be ignored. This is different from earlier behavior when a more complex stimulus (for example, a checkerboard) would be looked at longer than a simpler stimulus (a bull's eye, for instance). Kagan, who has been instrumental in the investigation of that period of life, feels these changes may suggest that discrepancy rather than complexity now begins to operate to control an infant's intentions (Kagan, 1971). This again suggests that the infant now can relate present experiences to previous happenings; that is, he or she makes use of early forms of memory.

10 to 18 months. Even the most casual observer of infants will stand in awe at the immense changes that take place in all developmental spheres during the second and third year of life. On the physical level we see the child's increasing mastery of his large muscles, beginning in stepping movements (40 weeks), the ability to stand alone (48 weeks), cruise (48 weeks), sit down voluntarily (52 weeks), and, finally, walk at 52 weeks. These developments, despite their immense importance for the infant's ability to become an individual in his own right by being able to move away from his mother, nevertheless are more or less refinements of patterns we saw first at 2 to 3 months when the baby could voluntarily raise his head. What is new at this age of about 10 months has to do with the way in which fine motor skills reflect advances in adaptive and social behavior. For example, at 40 weeks babies can release an object purposefully. They can also grasp a pellet at this time and a few weeks later put it into a bottle. They find a toy hidden behind a solid screen by 52 weeks, put a cube into a cup, imitate scribbling on paper, and begin to wave bye-bye. The imitative context in which these skills are learned is noteworthy. If a baby scribbles on a paper or waves bye-bye appropriately, he does so because someone in the family showed him. This implies that after 10 months, perceptual consequences are sought through imitation of fine motor and social behavior and not through the mere manipulation of objects as was done before. It is not surprising therefore that these new motor or biological skills go hand in hand with work on important personal and social developmental tasks that deal primarily with relationships with primary caretakers and the differentiation of self from others.

The gradual emergence of symbolic play is another aspect of development and can be observed towards the first birthday of an infant. While many of the imitative activities infants begin to engage in around 40 to 52 weeks are interpreted as play by parents, and indeed they are playful, it is only now that children can use toys to reflect something beyond the sensory motor experiences they present. For example, in play they will roll a car, put a bottle to a doll's face, and throw a ball, hence use toys in the way they are intended. This suggests that they have begun to generate hypotheses about how things work. This then gradually develops into pretence or symbolic play, first related to one's self (that is, a baby may pretend to comb her hair or drink out of an empty cup) and then to others (the baby will do these things to a doll). These simple play patterns will gradually become more complex; that is, children will substitute and change play sequences they have seen in others and create their own games and ideas.

By 6 months infants seem to ask what the object they have in their hands can do (for example, a rattle can make a certain noise) and will use the object accordingly. After 12 months, they seem to ask much more what they themselves can do with the toy in their hands (McCall, 1981). The older children get, the better they become in transforming one type of material into another. For example, at age 2 they will want to have real dolls or puppets to use as people in a domestic scene—while at 3 they may equally well use wooden blocks to represent people.

18 to 36 months. McCall (1981) states that the increasing predominance of verbal communication that characterizes the behavior of a child from 18 months onward marks this age as yet another time of specific developmental reorganization. Besides the infant's more skillful use of language in interacting with his or her environment, there occur other important events suggesting new and different mental realities and perspectives. Between 15 and 20 months infants begin to recognize themselves in the mirror (Amsterdam, 1972; Schulman & Kaplowitz, 1977) and to differentiate between themselves and others on photographs and videotapes (Lewis & Brooks-Gunn, 1979). This means that children have become aware of themselves as separate from others, a gigantic step in the consolidation of their humanness. It follows that children can now form their gender identity (Galenson & Roiphe, 1974), which is established during the second half of the second year, and that they will show very special responses to events that emotionally affect those to whom they feel close (Kagan, 1982). Other important changes within the "emotional" aspects of children's development at that time will be discussed in the next section.

The third year of life is characterized by the growing sophistication of the youngster's cognitive and motor skills. While by the age of 1 most children know three words, they have acquired some 300 by age 2 and 1000 by age 3. In concert with the increment of vocabulary, children during the late second and early third year of life learn how to think things through before they tackle a task. This allows them some sense of foresight. Likewise, they are able to conceptualize rules and regulations as they now have a better memory and can order things into all types of categories from big and small to right and wrong.

The ability to conceptualize the world in a concrete way and, to some extent, control it, also shows in the child's motor achievements. Children master feeding and dressing themselves and enjoy drawing and building things. They also, however, love to exercise their big muscles as seen in their beginning use of tricycles and jungle gym equipment.

In summary, we can see that children who approach their third birthday have experienced the emergence of all the basic ingredients of their future lives. They can use their bodies at will, are able to think independently though still concretely, have a basic notion of themselves and others, and have discovered the power of language. In later years they will use all these skills with far more sophistication and refinement. Yet nothing truly novel will be added to their cognitive and motor repertoire for the rest of their lives.

Emotional Development

Birth to 2 months. In the preceding section we said that a newborn infant's availability to the outside world depended upon his or her current state. A newborn who is in a quiet alert state will be able to take in and respond to his or her mother more differentially than one who is fussing or asleep. However, despite periods of obvious alertness, clinicians traditionally interested in the early emotional development of infants for many years postulated the presence of a "stimulus barrier" that was said to protect and isolate the infant against outside stimuli. The idea was that newborns were little fragments of living substance "suspended in the middle of an external world charged with the most powerful energies" (S. Freud, 1920/1950, p. 27). That is, they could not survive the strong external stimuli because of their immaturity and had to be shielded against them.

This theory of the potentially noxious stimuli coming from the outside world has been restated by many prominent psychoanalysts such as Rapaport (1951), Spitz (1961), and Mahler and McDevitt (1980) and has been quoted in support of the related concept that early infancy is an "autistic" experience (Mahler, Pine, & Bergmann, 1975). However, there is convincing evidence that even newborn infants will process information that has relevance, for example, to the attachment relationships they will develop with their primary caretakers. Before we give particular examples for this contention, it may be useful to discuss the concept of attachment in some more detail as it is one of the most crucial principles governing the development of children. Although the parent-child relationship is generally recognized as a dynamic dyad, that is, a system whose partners influence each other continuously, nevertheless theorists have oversimplified matters by analyzing this relationship primarily from the point of view of either one or the other of the participants. Thus the term "attachment" has generally been applied to the infant's behaviors, cognitions, and feelings toward his or her mother while the term "bonding" has been used to describe the mother's earliest feelings and behaviors toward her new infant.

As much of the work on attachment and bonding is based on Bowlby's theory of emotional development, we will first consider his account of common processes in the development of human attachment. Bowlby, a psychoanalyst and clinician by training, some 40 years ago became interested in studying the early relationships of children who became thieves in adolescence (Bowlby, 1944). He noticed that many of these youngsters seemed to show little concern for any other person and had never been closely attached to anyone during their lives. A significant number of these children had also experienced separations or other breaks in the relationships with their primary caretakers early in their lives. This led him to look at an infant's immediate reaction to his mother's disappearance and to conclude in 1951 that "what is to be essential for mental health is that the infant and young child should experience a warm, intimate and continuous relationship with his mother" (Bowlby, 1951, pp. 33-34). While Bowlby even today believes in the importance of this attachment relationship, his theory of the mechanisms of that relationship has developed substantially, as shown in his three volumes *Attachment* (1969), *Separation* (1973), and *Loss* (1980).

Bowlby sees attachment as a "system" composed of attachment behaviors that operate to keep the infant and mother in close proximity, as well as cognitions and affect that operate to organize and select these behaviors. The term "system" is used in the sense of a control system in engineering. Bowlby states that young infants in early history needed to be physically close to their mothers to be protected from potential outside dangers. This previously biological necessity, according to him, has now become instinctive in an ethological sense, that is, it is necessary for normal development to take place. For example, a smooth operation of the attachment system will allow other systems within the infant to predominate. If things go well the baby can expend his energies exploring the world around him rather than worrying about his mother's presence and his associated security. This in turn permits him to acquire new social and cognitive competence through interaction with this wider world and furthers his general development.

The organization of this attachment system during the first two months of life is steered primarily by the baby because his cognitive immaturity does not allow him to be very sensitive to minor changes in the caretaker's behavior patterns. However, his crying (Ainsworth, Blehar, Waters, & Walls, 1978), helplessness, and specific facial features

(Lorenz, 1950) seem to be destined to draw adults close to him and make it easier for them to treat him sensitively. In fact, Bowlby states the sensitivity of a mother or other caretaker to an infant's needs is the most important determinant of healthy emotional development (1969). It is interesting that experimental work by Ainsworth and her students (Ainsworth et al., 1978) has repeatedly confirmed the powerful correlation between maternal sensitivity and an infant's later feelings of security and well-being as shown by social competence and higher self-esteem.

Brazelton and his group (Brazelton, Tronick, Adamson, Als, & Wise, 1975) in an ingenious video double-screen design that allows the viewer to observe both the parent's and infant's faces simultaneously have shown that from 3 weeks onward infants show clear preference for human beings over objects. They also react in a characteristic way (for example, by looking away) to a human face that is immovable and still or that exhibits other distinct emotions such as sadness (Tronick, Ricks, & Cohn, 1982). This suggests that even newborn infants have an apparently inborn expectancy for interaction with their caretakers. These include a rhythmic cycling of attention and nonattention and the infant's apparent ability to perceive the internal laws governing similar concepts expressed through different sensory modalities. For example, an infant will remain calm if the mother makes a continuous sound and accompanies it with slow but continuous hand movements. If these same hand movements are presented with staccato type sounds, the infant will either look away or show his or her puzzlement through other behaviors (Stern, 1984). This function, which can also be shown across other modalities, is called "transmodal" behavior and is a basic paradigm of a relationship as it connects and synthesizes two or more apparently diverse phenomena. Furthermore, infants by 3 days discriminate between their mother's voice and that of another woman and will also work, by nonnutritive sucking, to produce their mother's voice in preference to the voice of another woman (DeCasper & Fifer, 1980). They also follow a human face for up to 80 degrees but will look at a garbled representation of a face much more briefly and follow it less (Goren, 1975). These abilities, which are not learned but clearly part of the infant's biological endowment, have been termed the infant's "prewired knowledge of the world" (Stern, Barnett, & Spieker, 1982). Their scientific charting has challenged many of the traditionally held beliefs of behaviorists and given some credibility to those who have insisted on the importance of very early experience for later development.

2 to 9 months. The emotional growth of an infant in this period is highlighted by the transformation from a primarily endogenously steered organism to a baby who very clearly responds to events around him or her. Initiated by the emergence of the social smile at about 6 weeks of age, infants now influence their environment not only through their instinctual and state behaviors (crying, smiling, startled, or mouthing movements) but also by their concrete reactions to their caretakers' behavior. This can be documented experimentally by the relative ease with which classical conditioning takes place. The infant, because of an improved state organization and prolonged alert states, can now direct more energy toward acquiring information from the outside world (Emde, Gaensbauer, & Harmon, 1976). This in turn allows a conditioned stimulus to acquire specific meaning and in that sense to become available for conditioning. The same maturational factors modify the attachment process. Although early on babies may show behavioral preference for their mothers over other women and may need her in close proximity in order to be reassured and secure, toward the end of this period they can also be calmed by the mother's voice from the adjacent room and even later by the "knowledge" that mom is somewhere in the house. In fact, Ainsworth and her students documented that infants whose mothers were relatively insensitive to their needs were insecure at 9 or 12 months. They would show this by ignoring or even physically attacking their mothers when they returned after a short separation (Ainsworth et al., 1978).

Despite the ability to conceptualize a mother's presence in a more sophisticated form at 9 or 12 months, the need for direct close physical contact with the primary caretaker will return whenever the infant becomes fearful or has other upsetting experiences. The ready and sensitive availability of the mother or other trusted caretakers therefore continues to be an important determinant of emotionally healthy growth.

Other behaviors of the baby that Bowlby calls "precursors to attachment" (1969) are the increasing signs that he or she prefers familiar over unfamiliar people. Mothers perceive their infants to show very distinct emotions as early as 3 months. In a study by Johnson, Dowling, and Wesner (1980), 100% of a sample of more than 600 mothers thought their babies showed interest and enjoyment, 69% surprise, 86% anger, and 69% fear. This suggests that parents develop very strong attributions about their young children's intentions and see them establishing an emotional signaling system very early in life

(Affleck, Tennen, & Gershman, 1984, April). It is not surprising, therefore, that 6-month-old infants will look and smile, touch or coo— that is, use all their multiple sensory modalities—to engage and respond to their mothers far more than strangers. The range or depth of the feelings expressed by the baby likewise increase during this time. The infant who at 3 months, when dissatisfied, may simply cry or turn away, will have, at 8 months, developed easily understood affective facial expressions or body postures to communicate his or her disapproval actively.

Finally, the attachment to the caregiver during these months also becomes a mode through which the infant can overcome and weather stresses. A mother or father can now "rescue" and calm an upset or frightened baby with the help of an individually established style of interaction. Such an experience of being repeatedly calmed by mother or father will help the infant to develop a sense of confidence and trust and build up a feeling that the world is a place that will turn out to be safe in the end; that is, it helps him or her to build up resilience.

Most parents almost automatically echo or "mirror" what the infant does when they play with him or her (Papousek & Papousek, 1979) and in that way provide a natural contingency. Thus parents will repeat sounds the baby makes and engage in many intricate affective inter-changes (Call, 1980; Stern, 1983), which all help the infant to feel as a valued individual.

The process of differentiation, that is, the ability to separate one person from another or to experience how one can effect changes in the environment, occurs in all the infant's realms of experience (Emde et al., 1976; Stern, 1974). It gradually brings about an awareness of the causality of life's phenomena, the power one has to influence them, and thereby it forms one source of the child's self-esteem. An environment that does not read the infant's signals or is unable to respond differentially to them may well inhibit normal growth and compromise the development of later coping strategies.

10 to 18 months. As the infant becomes more expert in differentiating means from ends, this learning about the relationship between events and their consequences seems to know no bounds. The early toddler shows increasingly more imitative behaviors, which in turn facilitate exploration and learning of new connections between his or her feelings and environmental actions. He or she also practices his or her newly acquired skills as they pertain to his or her body. He or she will crawl, climb, and move about with great pleasure and will gradually learn to detach himself or herself from his or her mother and other main caretakers. This process, one of the paramount steps in development, Mahler, Pine, and Bergmann (1975) have called the "separation-individuation" process. The process begins at around 7 months when infants begin to crawl away from mother, use more distant means of communication (for instance, looking rather than touching), discover the peek-a-boo game, and spend much time exploring their caretaker's face and body. This phase lasts 4 to 5 months, and Mahler calls it the "differentiation phase."

From 10 to about 15 months the baby appears to practice endlessly the physical separation from his or her primary caretakers by joyously running away from them. At other times, however, the infant becomes very anxious as he or she can now realize that the world contains all kinds of potential dangers and that a life away from his or her mother is fraught with pitfalls and difficulties. Hence this "practicing phase" of the child's newly discovered independence contains both positive and negative aspects of behavior. Anger that formerly was discharged diffusely now also becomes more focused and directed against the parent. It looks as if at times the infant is furious at his or her relative impotence vis-à-vis the world and can only take charge of it by refusing to obey its laws and regulations. Thus much of this phase of exploration can only proceed smoothly if the caretakers are emotionally available to the child. Such availability is tested out by the child through frequent looks at his or her mother, referred to as "emotional referencing" (Bowlby, 1969; Matas, Arend, & Sroufe, 1978). In a recent study Sorce and Emde (1981) have found that 15-month-old children when exposed to a new and unusual toy (an R_2D_2 robot from the *Star Wars* trilogy) would not explore the robot. They would often hide behind a chair when their mothers were in the same room but reading, while the children were physically far more active in exploring the robot when their mother simply looked at them.

A similar phenomenon, termed "social referencing" (Klinnert et al., 1982), has been described by members of Emde's research team. These workers found that infants will look at their caretakers to seek out emotional information when confronting an event they could not make sense of on their own. The parents responded in such a situation by guiding the infant's immediate action; for example, they would lead him or her either to cross a certain threshold on a plexiglass-covered table or turn around and crawl away from it. This suggests that the emotional signaling system of infants has become extremely sophisticated by this time and that adequate and sensitive responding of caretakers will provide important ingredients for healthy emotional and social development.

18 to 36 months. This period is highlighted by the final episode of Mahler's separation-individuation process. Beginning at about 18 months and extending to 24 months, toddlers seem to realize and accept that there are many things they cannot yet do, but that there are also definite tasks that they have mastered. Thus children will proudly and competently feed themselves now, get dressed, play out concerns they have in their games, and in many ways present a far more solid sense of separateness. This shows itself in fewer tantrums and somewhat less confrontational behavior toward the parents. Thus Mahler calls this the period of "rapprochement."

At the same time infants become aware of their gender, learn to name other parts of their bodies, respond to their own mirror images, and have an increasingly clear concept of their mothers and fathers.

During the ensuing months both boys and girls will continue to practice their newly found identity and try out others as well. Thus they will want to play various roles such as father, mother, doctor, or nurse and will often begin to do this in the company of other children their age. Boys will sporadically dress in girls' clothing and girls will want to urinate standing up. Boys in general will show a far greater amount of outward aggression at this time (Maccoby & Jacklin, 1974), although the fantasies of all toddlers seem to be filled with destructive fears and wishes such as wicked witches who eat children and then get burned. While some girls will show a distinct sadness about not having a penis and both boys and girls are preoccupied with their sexual organs and their meaning and function (Galenson & Roiphe, 1974), there is no evidence that concern about anatomical differences between the sexes usually leads to later problems.

SUMMARY

The preceding two chapters have exposed us to some of the more important developmental changes seen in children during the first three years of life. In addition to the behavioral data on which we base our theoretical concepts of development, we have also touched on some more controversial issues of development, such as the degree of continuity and discontinuity we see in development, the evidence we have in support of particular theories of development, and the degree to which either emotional, biological, or cognitive factors are the precursors needed for developmental change.

What we hope we have demonstrated in discussing these various issues are (1) the changes that take place in the field of academic developmental psychology and psychiatry at this very time and (2) the enormous complexity of the developmental process. We have undoubtedly also shown that we do not yet have an all-encompassing theory of child development, although more professionals are working on the construction of better theoretical models than ever before.

4

PSYCHIATRIC ASSESSMENT OF INFANTS AND THEIR FAMILIES

In a psychiatric assessment of infants, clinicians aim to obtain a data base that allows them to come to a diagnostic understanding of both infants and the people who care for them. The information clinicians obtain should also allow them to say something about the likely future course of any condition at hand and help them in planning appropriate and specific interventions.

Assessing infants and their families requires particular skills and sensitivities. The reasons for this are related on the one hand to the very special needs of infants that bind them to their caretakers and therefore make them understandable only within this interactive system. On the other hand, they are characterized by a complex network of functions reflecting their biological, cognitive, and socioemotional endowments and needs. Clinicians must learn about the strengths and vulnerabilities of these functions and must be able to elicit and to demonstrate them to the caregivers. To be experts in diagnosing difficulties, clinicians must also be experts on normal child development.

Finally, clinicians must be able to assess both positive and negative aspects of an infant's caretaking situation in detail. They will usually aim to enhance the caretaking abilities of those living with the infant patient and must achieve that goal within a spirit of partnership and cooperation.

Despite these age-specific precautions, the clinicians who work with infants will use many of the skills they have learned with older populations. The present chapter, after briefly discussing general interviewing techniques, will review these "ordinary" assessment skills and give an outline of the data that should be collected on children and families of all ages. We will then describe in more detail those parts of an assessment that are specific to infancy and require particular techniques.

INTERVIEWING TECHNIQUES

There is good evidence that various interviewing styles will elicit very similar information from the parents of young patients. However, recent studies have shown that factual historical data may best be obtained by direct questions (Cox, Hopkinson, & Rutter, 1981). Feelings and opinions, in contrast, are elicited more easily when the interviewer asks open questions such as "What does he do when you go away?" or uses inferences or interpretation (for example, "This must have reminded you of your father's anger at you") or linkages ("Having him cry all the time must have made you feel sad"; Hopkinson, Cox, & Rutter, 1981). Such indirect and synthesizing remarks are most likely helpful because they suggest to parents that they have been understood, that the interviewer shares their sentiments, and that the interviewer can therefore be trusted.

Two of the most common reasons for an unsatisfactory interview are

(1) the clinician's poor interviewing techniques and
(2) the clinician's conceptual limitations related to psychiatric theory and practice.

Here are some examples of poor interviewing techniques. Interviewers should not ask a parent more than one question at the same time, nor should they ask multiple-choice questions (for example, "Does he get angry because of X, Y, or Z?"). Because none of the suggested answers may be correct, parents may feel loath to say so.

Interviewers should also not accept a parent's jargon without asking for clarification (for instance, "He feels bad when I come near him"). In that case it is not clear what the parent means by the word "bad."

Finally, it is usually not helpful to ask direct or closed questions (such as, "How often does he wet the bed?") or to let the interview ramble on unchecked without providing any structure. In these cases the interviewer may be unable to tap emotional issues or else go on too long.

Problems related to conceptual limitations often occur when clinicians avoid broaching personal issues out of fear of upsetting the parent or when they fail to pick up leads given by the parent, such as a change in mother's speech rhythm, a glance toward the husband, or a change of topic or of a parent's pitch of voice. An interviewer's hesitation to pursue a topic with more detailed questions, such as the quality of the marital relationship, likewise often leads to poor and incomplete histories. Finally, the belief that people can have only one disorder or *either* an emotional *or* a physical problem may bring about the premature closure of an interview and result in an incomplete data base.

OUTLINE OF ASSESSMENT DATA

Remember that the information you obtain from any patient or his or her caretakers must be divided into factual data—such as age, sex, and the dates of illnesses—and opinions. The latter may be more or less distorted reflections of reality as seen by the infant's parents. Nevertheless, opinions are often important parameters that allow clinicians to understand an infant's life space. However, they must be assessed and recorded with their necessary limitations in mind.

Likewise, a psychiatric history should be made up of factual information—encompassing data about the family, the identified patient and his or her particular condition—as well as clinical opinions. Such opinions are usually expressed in the formulation of the case. Clinicians here try to make sense of the variety of data presented to them by adding a personal judgment to the story of Jane or John. Their judgment often reflects their own values and may be disputed by others who, using the same factual data base, may formulate very different opinions the validity of which only time may judge.

The factual data base of a psychiatric assessment should include identifying data, reason for referral, history of current difficulties, family history, developmental history, and the clinician's assessment of the infant.

Identifying Data

These data should include the patient's and caretakers' name, address, telephone number, age, sex, race, and legal status of the child (for instance, natural child, adopted or foster).

Reason for Referral

A description of the reason for referral should include a short description of concerns and the person(s) who hold them and their reasons.

History of Current Difficulties

The history describes the patient's problem(s), their detailed course and severity, how they were first noted, possible precipitating events, what makes problems worse and better, what caretakers and others have done to help and what has been achieved, and how the family or other important caretakers understand the problem(s).

Family History

(1) The family history should have data on the parents' and/or present caretakers' personal life experiences. This includes information about the parenting they received, possible separation and illnesses they experienced, their educational or occupational careers, any familial medical or psychiatric conditions and their own medical history, quality and type of past and present relationships with their own parents, siblings, and peers, as well as the patient's siblings.

(2) The siblings' identifying data and personal life experiences. This includes any separations they have had from primary caretakers and their reactions to them, the presence of illnesses, and their relationship to the identified patient.

(3) Data on other important caretakers (or caretaking institutions) of the infant such as grandparents, babysitters, daycare center personnel, professionals within the court system, or children's aid societies, and their sensitivity to the infant's needs.

Developmental History

This includes a detailed exploration of all developmental aspects of the biological, cognitive, and socioemotional life of the infant. Areas to be covered should include:

(1) Physical, cognitive, and emotional milestones: when did the baby first sit, stand, walk, or ride a tricycle; his or her first smile, first recognition of

himself or herself as a separate person; stranger anxiety; when did he or she become aware of being a boy or a girl; the child's use of the form "I" when talking about himself or herself; and responding to others' feelings.

(2) A detailed description of the pregnancy and the infant's neonatal period: this should, if possible, include information about the mother's fantasies about the baby during her pregnancy, her feelings during the birth, and the behavior of others such as the obstetrician or her husband during that time; inquire also about the mother's initial impressions of the baby, as well as the baby's early reactions toward her and others (for instance, was he or she cuddly, interested, or sleepy?).

(3) The infant's early behavioral organization: could the baby be consoled easily—and what methods had to be used; could the baby console himself or herself and how was that achieved; what was the infant's general activity level, how regular was he or she in sleeping, walking, and eating; how adaptable and reactive was the child to new stimuli and how able to attend to his or her surroundings?

(4) Degree of individuation from family such as general level of independence or involvement with peers or nursery school personnel.

(5) Special strengths and vulnerabilities, that is, musical or other talents; shyness or sensitivities to particular events such as meeting new people, loud noises, being offered a new food; vulnerability to specific physical illnesses.

(6) Response to previous stresses such as medical illnesses, parental absence, the move to a new house or apartment, or the birth of a sibling.

More detailed expositions of a standard psychiatric evaluation of a child and his or her family can be obtained in the regular textbooks of child psychiatry (see Cohen, 1979; Lewis, 1982; Steinhauer & Rae-Grant, 1983). The interviewer should finally always be aware that mothers, despite the emotional meaning the early life of an infant has to them, are only moderately good historians (Minde, Webb, & Sykes, 1968). Thus they frequently recall even direct historical data incorrectly and change their interpretation of past events in line with the perceived present difficulties of the baby. For example, a mother is more likely to label an infant as having been temperamentally difficult all his or her life if her present complaints are around his or her constant crying or irritability.

The Clinical Infant Assessment

Assessment of infants is best done through a comprehensive developmental diagnostic process. This includes an initial interview with the parents or other primary caretakers, developmental testing of the child, and play interviews.

(1) Initial interview with the parents or other primary caretakers.
This interview should be held without the baby or young child to acquire
background data on both the child and his or her family as outlined in
the previous section. It should be stressed that the interview is not only a
source for gathering information but also a time during which the
clinician can observe the interaction of the parents with each other, their
understanding and sensitivity to the child, and their conceptualization
of development in general. The relationship can be assessed initially by
seeing which parent gives which part of the history and how that is done
and whether there are disagreements in the parents' opinions about the
child's symptoms or life experiences and how they are solved. One may
also ask directly how the parents share their caretaking role and how
supported or isolated they feel from each other. While the intricacies of
the human relationship are clearly beyond the scope of an initial
interview, there is good evidence that one can get a reliable estimate of
the overall marital harmony by examining parental cooperation on
everyday concrete tasks (Brown & Rutter, 1966). Questions here would
deal with such issues as the number of times the husband helps his wife
with the dishes, the frequency with which they go out to a movie, and
so on.

The parental understanding of the infant's present condition obviously varies enormously. Factors that contribute to this variation may
be the parental conceptualization of development as a whole. For
example, some parents see infants to be either good or bad, tend to have
a very biological outlook on development, and do not see a child's
present state as the synthesis of environmental and biological forces
(Sameroff & Chandler, 1975). Other families look for recent changes in
the child's life space to evaluate his or her functions and may, through
using particular attributions, experience a great deal of guilt, anxiety, or
helplessness. It is therefore important to find out about these issues early
on and stress the parents' expert knowledge of their child as well as the
help the clinician will need to have from them. Parental concepts or
attributions to normal or abnormal development are also related
importantly to later treatment suggestions; parents who feel personally
responsible for their child's developmental progress are generally more
open to therapeutic interventions than are those who view life as a
predetermined chain of events (Affleck, Tennen, & Gershman, 1984).

(2) Developmental testing of the child. After the parent interview the
child is seen for a general developmental assessment. This ideally takes

place in a specially equipped room in the presence of one or both parents. Their presence is important not only to comfort and reassure the young child in a new place but also to allow the parent to see how the child performs on the tasks given by the examiner.

The value of this can be twofold. The examiner will demonstrate the strengths and/or weaknesses of the child's performance and so help the parents to come to a more realistic perception of their infant's abilities (Field, 1982). Parents will also witness and partake in a sensitive interchange between their youngster and another adult. Such an encounter can potentially teach them something about the way one might interact with one's child and possibly also be an introduction to ways that may modify or at least manage particular behavioral deviations. Shared observations also facilitate later communication of the diagnostic formulation by the clinician.

The parents' presence in the test situation also allows the examiner a view of the parent-child interaction. Facets of this interaction may center around the parents' ability and/or wish to provide emotional support for the child and their possible intrusiveness into the testing and their reactions to displays of particular behaviors of the child toward the examiner.

The number of appointments necessary to complete the evaluation depends on the child's attentiveness, physical status, and motivation. In our experience two sessions of 40 to 45 minutes' duration will usually be sufficient.

The routine tests we find most useful at this stage of the assessment are contained in the Yale Developmental Schedules developed by Provence and her colleagues at the Yale Study Center (Provence, Leonard, & Naylor, 1982). The Yale schedules consist of items for children aged 4 weeks to 6 years. They come from the Gesell, Merrill-Palmer, Stanford-Binet, and Hetzer-Wolf tests from the Viennese Scale. The test protocol has been used for more than 30 years by Provence and her group, and while the individual test items are standardized, the composite protocol has never been formally validated. The items provide an estimate of the child's current level of functioning in various areas. Categories assessed by these schedules include gross motor, fine motor, adaptive, language, and personal-social behavior. Gross motor items measure large muscle skills. Fine motor items assess finger and hand skills. Adaptive items assess primarily nonverbal problem-solving ability, imitation, and manipulation of objects. Language items measure both receptive and expressive language and can be used to reveal a child's capacity for symbolic thought and fantasy.

While the test protocol is used to obtain a general idea of the child's developmental status, in each of the five sections in which the items are arranged, the testing has two other equally important functions. It is a structured situation in which we can assess the quality as much as the quantity of the child's work. How does 2-year-old Danny react when he does not know an answer—can he rejoice when he has mastered the task? How does he cope or compensate for apparent shortcomings? Can he relate to the examiner as a trustworthy person or does he see him as an adversary? The test also serves as an excellent assessment of the child's general neurological integration. One can assess the muscle strength, tone, and symmetry and coordination and ease of movements. In that way the clinician can gain more useful information about the central nervous system (CNS) functioning than during a conventional neurological examination. Other behavioral functions normally subsumed under the mental status examination—such as attention span, modulation of impulse, the ability to organize material and activities— can also be observed during the testing sessions and often add very significant diagnostic data. For more stringently validated infant tests, the reader is referred to the following chapter.

A further major advantage of beginning the evaluation with the developmental schedules described above is that this allows the children to form a relationship with the examiner by "doing things" with him or her, which most of them find interesting. This is compatible with the various themes of the preschooler's existence—that of experimenting, exploring, and being active. The adults' participation in such activities, therefore, is far less threatening for a young child than being with a strange new grownup person who quickly tries to learn things about defences and secret feelings. In fact, our clinical experience suggests that the play sessions that follow a developmental assessment have a far richer quality as both partners know each other already and the clinician can use these sessions to probe into areas still unclear to him or her in a more goal-directed fashion.

(3) Play interviews. Children of about 18 months of age or older are seen for two or three play sessions after the testing sessions. Younger infants may not require more than one such session. Play interviews are generally unstructured sessions during which the young child can choose freely what to play and do. Toys offered to a child should cover a wide range of themes. There should be some dolls representing a family

and other people, animal puppets, preferably a doll's house with furniture, a few small cars, dishes, cutlery, and plasticine. It is important to have some potentially frightening animals such as a lion or tiger among the cows, sheep, and pigs and also to have puppets that represent authority or danger (such as a policeman or fireman). We also always try to have two guns, two telephones, and a doctor's kit in the playroom so that the clinician can be an active partner in the play sequence.

It is essential for children under 3 that most of the toys look realistic as their sense of abstraction and their ability to engage in symbolic play are not yet sufficiently developed to use, for example, a block for a telephone or a car.

From the play sessions the clinician can usually make inferences about the child's inner life: his or her conflicts, desires, fears, and wishes and their possible source. The clinician can also assess the child's coping strategies, defensive functions, modes of affective expression, and his or her ability to form a relationship with the examiner.

It should be stressed that such diagnostic play is different from the general play the clinician may engage in with children in therapy since the purpose is investigative. For example, during therapy the clinician may want to stop or intervene when John repeatedly plays out a gruesome mass murder scene because the clinician wants to reinforce the concept of a caring and regulated environment. However, during an assessment play period, the clinician may simply comment that all the people and animals get killed here but not attempt automatically to calm an overexcited, screeching youngster.

Play sessions for infants under 18 months consist mainly in observing spontaneous play with toys and engaging them in games such as peek-a-boo or pat-a-cake. While the ability of young infants to play symbolically is still not well developed, they nevertheless will exhibit a wide range of behaviors both toward their parents and the clinician, providing important information about their concept of our world and their general comfort or discomfort with it.

THE ASSESSMENT OF PARENTING SKILLS

One of the most difficult parts of the psychiatric assessment is the evaluation of the caretaker's ability to meet the young child's developmental needs. The reasons for this are multiple since caretaking is made up of many different tasks and requirements. These range on one level from providing basic shelter, food, and warmth to an infant, to giving him or her a carefully balanced diet and a bed of his or her own in a clean house. Another dimension could range from recognizing that children are not merely small adults but need some emotional consideration to participate with genuine pleasure in the little games with which an infant attempts to challenge the world. Further complexities in measuring parenting abilities arise because the mother who may be "good enough," to use a phrase of Winnicott (1960), in her care during the first 6 months of a child's life—who enjoys the seemingly unlimited giving of comfort to the young infant—may resent this same infant's increasing demands for separation and individuation later on. Children are also differentially equipped to cope with a marginal environment and some may "make do" while others wither helplessly. The phenomenon of discontinuity in development outlined in Chapter 2 can also work for or against a given child. For example, an older child, by becoming mobile and having acquired language, may find substitute sources of stimulation and aids to cognitive growth that were not accessible to the younger infant.

Another kind of problem is presented by those infants who in response to traumatic biological or emotional life events require very special ways of handling, not usually part of a mother's repertoire of caretaking practices. Here a failure to provide developmentally appropriate caretaking may reflect the parents' ignorance of knowing the "right way" of handling the child rather than be symptomatic of their particular psychological or psychosocial limitations. Finally, caretakers vary not only in their specific strengths but also in their day-to-day competence.

What then should we look for in parents of young children when we assess their parenting competence? We suggest that parents be rated on five general and relatively stable dimensions that contribute to their interpersonal interactions regardless of the child's developmental stage. These dimensions are derived from the writings of Provence, Leonard, and Naylor (1982); Anna Freud (1965); Rutter and associates (1975); Ainsworth and associates (1978); and Ramey, Bryant, Sparling, and Wasik (1984); and they have roots within both the psychoanalytic and behavioral traditions of child development.

Parental Rating

General ratings. During an interview parents should be rated on their

(1) general emotional and physical health,
(2) self-esteem,
(3) general coping and adaptation skills,
(4) authoritarian versus democratic attitudes, and
(5) willingness and/or ability to provide developmental encouragement.

The assessment of the parents' past and present emotional and physical health has been discussed in an earlier section of this chapter. It is important to remember, however, that many parents bring their emotional problems to the attention of general practitioners rather than mental health specialists. Hence an examiner should always ask whether mother or father take "nerve pills" or talked to their GP about "special problems." The Malaise Inventory, a 20-item questionnaire developed by Rutter (1970) from items of the Cornell Medical Index, is a useful tool in assessing physical manifestations of parental anxiety, depression, or abnormal thought processes.

Self-esteem can often only be estimated from incidental statements of the parents. For example, a mother may say, "Michael doesn't listen to me—nor does anyone else in the family"; a father may remark, "I would be so happy if Evelyn would smile at me just once a week." Both of these statements may be reflections of a low self-esteem and should alert the clinician to search for other signs of self-deprecation.

General coping and adaptation skills can be assessed by inquiring how previous stresses have been managed, which will often be reported quite accurately by parents when they are directly asked about them. Remember that there are many ways to cope with difficulties, ranging from complete denial to active working through. The final rating of coping skills should be based on the effectiveness of these strategies rather than on the type of defense or coping mechanism used.

Authoritarian or democratic attitudes can be assessed by evaluating the decision-making process in a family. Few families function in a totally authoritarian or democratic mode, and in many families specific interaction patterns work well. The clinician's judgment must always take this into consideration.

The willingness to provide developmental encouragement does not only refer to the parents' ability to "stimulate" an infant. In fact, parents can be withdrawn and unavailable but also intrusive and hyperstimulating or shifting between the two modalities. Both extremes tend to be maladaptive and may undermine the infant's phase-expected capacities.

In addition to these general ratings we have also found it useful to inquire about the routines of an average day of the infant and his or her family. This can provide us with a sense of the stresses the family faces and also gives us the possibility of assessing the family's support systems and child-rearing attitudes which is yet another way to evaluate their degree of developmental encouragement.

We also observe the caretakers' response to us as professionals and as people, noting their predominant mood and thinking style. Such observations can help us predict the parents' readiness and/or ability to engage with us in a therapeutic teaching process and may forecast our chance of influencing the parent-infant interaction.

Specific Parameters

Keeping in mind the important qualitative changes that infants undergo during the first 3 years in their development requiring variable types of nurturing experiences, we suggest that in addition to the previously mentioned general parameters of parenting, the following skills are essential for good parenting during specific developmental stages.

(1) The ability to help the child in organizing his or her behavior. This ability is of special importance for newborn infants as their adaptive self-regulatory capacities provide them with the first experience of tension release and some form of mastery over the world. Parents can help in making this capacity more adaptive by learning about the individual characteristics of their babies and by building on their strength to aid them to achieve harmony and regulation. In practice this may mean that parents have a sense of little Janie's preferred sleeping position, the way she should be held and calmed, and the position most

conducive to interesting her in the world. The clinician may also want to assess how parents even at an early stage allow her to lead her transactions with the world—whether they give her time to move her head or make a sound and repeat it rather than try to tickle her awake and then expect her to respond appropriately. The benefit of an imitative parental interaction over more invasive patterns has been well established by Field (1977).

In the case of infants who because of a biological or genetic insult have a decreased capacity for self-regulation, the parents' ability to soothe and regulate the infant's behavior may be more difficult but also far more important for the infant's future development. In assessing these skills we have found it useful to differentiate between caretakers who respond inappropriately because they do not see or experience the needs of a child and those who perceive these needs but cannot act because of personal problems or limitations. Some parents may also show a transient inability to perceive and/or respond to their children's needs because of fatigue or other environmental stresses, and the accurate diagnosis of such a pattern is obviously important.

(2) Sensitivity and availability of the primary caretaker. It can be said that good parenting is the sensitive appraisal of a child's inner and outer needs and the provision of those needs through developmentally relevant channels. However, we feel that the emotional availability of a mother or her substitute is especially important during the second quarter of the infant's first year because of the developing attachment system. A baby falls in love with his or her caretakers during this time, and the environment's role in making that come about cannot be overemphasized. Clinically this may best be shown by the parents' pleasure in being with the baby, the depth and range of all affects shown, and their joy in the infant's increasing ability to reciprocate their feelings. It will also be reflected in the parents' ability to understand and sympathize with the infant when he or she wants to be left alone or change a particular type of interaction. In growth-promoting families we will also witness the beginning of private games between mothers and their babies, all marking the development of a personal style of parent-infant attachment.

(3) Contingent behavior. The word "contingency" implies the caretaker's rapid response to his or her baby's expressed needs and desires. In comparison to the sensitive parent, the contingent parent is one who will respond rapidly and exclusively to his or her infant's requests. Such rapid responses during the second to fourth quarter of the first year have been found to be highly correlated with an infant's secure attachment to his or her mother later on in life (Ainsworth et al., 1978) and with the amount and quality of interactions between medically compromised infants and their parents (Minde, Marton, Manning, & Hines, 1980). This suggests that most contingent mothers are also sensitive to their children.

Clinicians can assess clinically the parents' contingency by inquiring about their attitude and response to the infant's crying. Parents who respond immediately when their young infant is upset are highly contingent in their behaviors. There is no evidence that such rapid responding leads to later "spoiling" (Bell & Ainsworth, 1972) as crying during the first year is an attempt to communicate genuine needs, which, when satisfied quickly, will teach the baby that the world is a place where one can be relieved of bad feelings without undue delay.

(4) Stimulation. The variety, spontaneity, and richness of an environment has long been seen as a vital ingredient of a child's later emotional and cognitive functioning (Birch & Gussow, 1970; Deutsch, 1964; Ramey, MacPhee, & Yates, 1982). Recent studies also show that it is especially from the second year of life onward that an environment which provides multiple types of play material, permits visual and physical exploration (Wachs, 1978, 1979), and makes available a stimulus shelter where the child can escape for quiet moments alone (Gottfried & Gottfried, 1984) becomes the best predictor of the child's later functioning. It must be emphasized that intellectual stimulation appears to be most effective if it arises out of the joint play with a caregiver or is protectively structured for the child by somebody for whom he or she cares (Carew, 1980; Clarke-Stewart, 1973). This means that an assessment of the stimulation value of a home environment can best be done by learning how much the parent or other caretaker plays with his or her child, what their games consist of and how age-appropriate this stimulation is, and parents' discernment about when to participate actively, when to provide support from a distance, and when

to leave a child to his or her own devices. Stimulation is evaluated as a means of helping the child feel that he can master things and develop a sense of effectance (White, 1959; Yarrow, Rubenstein, & Pederson, 1975).

A related concept that has been found to be a major building block in creating this sense of mastery is the caretaker's ability or willingness to provide a social "scaffold" for the child's learning experiences (Bruner, 1978), especially as it relates to joint attention and joint action. For example, in the peek-a-boo game the mother first hides and then uncovers herself, while later the child does the hiding and uncovering (Bruner & Sherwood, 1976). Similarly, mothers play very different games with 6- and 12-month-old children (Gustafson, Green, & West, 1979). Early games are typically geared to the infant's more passive role (bouncing), while later roll-the-ball or peek-a-boo games stress the active role the child can take in these interactions. A recent study by Hodapp, Goldfield, and Boyatzis (1984) gives a very good illustration of these issues. Hodapp observed 17 mother-infant pairs (babies between the ages of 8 and 16 months) once a month and asked the mothers to play a number of common games with their children. During the early months when the child could not yet return the ball in the roll-a-ball game, mothers spent a good deal of time (57%) in getting the infant's attention and setting the stage (repositioning the child, cleaning obstacles out of the way, and so on) for the game (46%). Once the infant began to roll the ball back, however, these behaviors decreased significantly (to 41% and 17% respectively). How important these mutual games are for general development was shown by the fact that these children gave back objects to the experimenter in a formal testing situation a full 1.7 months later than they had returned them to their mothers during the game.

These data imply that mothers scaffold the acquisition of skills in their children by first constraining the free variation of their infant's behavior (through stage setting and getting attention) and then channeling their approximations of a new skill into its optimal form (by holding out hands, leaning forward, encouraging, and so on). It is obvious that the specific scaffolding practices that most mothers perform seemingly automatically (Papousek & Papousek, 1979) will vary with the development of the infant. However, their presence seems to reflect an important aspect of sensitive mothering and should be part of the mother-infant evaluation.

Other Evaluations

The reader may have noticed that the assessment process discussed in the present chapter was geared toward the infant who has normal or slightly abnormal cognitive abilities. For infants who show specific developmental aberrations, special medical, neurological, or psychological evaluations may have to be suggested. While the present text cannot go into the details of all available medical or psychological procedures, the following chapter will discuss a number of psychological tests that may be helpful in a more detailed assessment.

SUMMARY

In this chapter we have examined the basic variables that make up an evaluation of an infant or young child and his or her family. It is clear that the various types of information obtained must now be integrated into the story of Anna, Betty, or Carl. No test or interaction observation can ever be put to clinical use without this synthesis of all the data. The final summary or formulation should also address the strengths and weaknesses of the family, the child and its social matrix, the family's expectations of the clinician's assessment and possible treatment and list those factors that may perpetuate the present problems or help to eliminate them.

5

INFANT TESTING

Psychological tests are valued by clinicians and researchers as systematic procedures for the observation and description of behavior. Infant mental health professionals can choose from a wide range of tests designed to assist them in identifying children with problems in different areas of development, in making decisions about specific treatments or special care, and in monitoring their developmental status over time. Thus tests can play a significant role in the care of infants, and it is therefore important to know how to use them. This chapter has two objectives: to give an overview of infant tests and to make the test user aware of the problems inherent in testing infants.

PROBLEMS OF INFANT TESTS

A standardized assessment that uses "measures," "scales," or "instruments" and summarizes the results in the form of numerical scores conveys the notion that testing is an exact science that supplies us with hard data and scientific information. This is not the case. Regardless of the relative excellence of any particular test, tests are not infallible. Among the reasons for this are problems related to the reliability and validity of a test as well as the very nature of the individual organism or behavior under study.

THE PROBLEM OF TEST RELIABILITY

Reliability is generally referred to as the consistency of scores the same individuals obtain when reexamined with the same test on different occasions (test-retest reliability), or by different examiners (interexaminer, interrater, or interobserver reliability). Both are important considerations for the test developer. In general, an infant test should have a high interexaminer reliability, that is, items should be clearly worded, and they should refer to distinct behaviors so that well-trained examiners observing the same performance achieve a high degree of agreement in their rating.

The test user also needs to bear in mind that the consistency of scores depends on the ability of the subject or patient to produce the same response reliably. Young children are notoriously variable in this respect. Their responses may vary according to changes in state, for example, whether they are hungry, tired, teething, alert, or full of energy. Their responses may also depend on how comfortable they feel in the testing situation, which may be at home or in the clinic, with or without the regular caretaker present, with a familiar or unfamiliar examiner. Another important variable is the kind of rapport the test administrator is able to achieve. As Uzgiris and Hunt (1975) remind us, a rating of "no response" or "no interest" may be more due to a lack of coordination between the intentions of the infant and those of the examiner than to a lack of capability on the part of the infant. This problem may be partly overcome by assuring that the examiner is not only well-trained in the mechanics of the particular test, but that he or she has experience in dealing with infants and is sensitive to variations in their mood and behavior. The younger the child, the more difficult it is for the examiner to control the testing situation by instructions. Thus it is the "guile" of the examiner, in addition to the inherent interest of the test items, that is critical to successful testing (Yang, 1979; Yarrow & Pedersen, 1976).

Another point that has to be considered is the phenomenon of development itself, which defies the notion of stability that psychometricians used to demand. Thus, while we should look for high intertester reliability, we should not be overly concerned with the comparatively low test-retest reliability reported for many infant tests, especially where younger infants and greater test-retest intervals are concerned. There are new statistical aids available to deal with the problem of dependability of measurements, well discussed by Messick (1983).

THE PROBLEM OF TEST VALIDITY

The two types of validity that are of major interest to the user of infant tests are *concurrent validity*, which refers to the degree to which

TABLE 5.1
Median Correlations Across Studies Between
Infant Test Scores and Childhood IQ

Age of Childhood Test (years)	Age of Infant Test (months)				
	1-6	7-12	13-18	19-30	
8-18	0.06 (6/4)	0.25 (3/3)	0.32 (4/3)	0.49 (34/6)	0.28
5-7	0.09 (6/4)	0.20 (5/4)	0.34 (5/4)	0.39 (13/5)	0.25
3-4	0.21 (16/11)	0.32 (14/12)	0.50 (9/7)	0.59 (15/6)	0.40
	0.12	0.26	0.39	0.49	

SOURCE: McCall (1979, p. 712). Reprinted by permission of the author and John Wiley & Sons, Inc.
NOTE: Decimal entries indicate median correlation, the numbers in parentheses give the number of different r's and the number of independent studies used to calculate the median. In the case of more than one r per study, the median r for that study was entered into the calculation of the cell median. Marginal values indicate the average of the median r's presented in that row or column.

test results accurately portray the current level of functioning, and *predictive validity*, which refers to the extent to which current test results predict future functioning. As might be inferred from the above, concurrent validity depends not only on characteristics of the test itself but also on the ability of the examiner to elicit the relevant behaviors from the infant, as well as on the infant's ability or motivation to produce a response that is representative of his or her current status. While it is difficult to ascertain the concurrent validity of an infant measure in the absence of appropriate objective criteria, it is possible for an individual examiner to make this judgment about the performance of an individual infant, if he or she can draw on additional information, such as maternal reports, independent observations, or a retest under different circumstances.

Even if high concurrent validity of a measure were established beyond any doubt, this by itself should not necessarily guarantee its predictive validity. In fact, with regard to developmental tests, it has consistently been found that there is virtually no relationship between early test scores and cognitive performance in later childhood. Only after the first 18 months of life do instruments predict later intelligence to any practical extent. This is well illustrated in Table 5.1.

Indeed, as McCall (1979) observed, prediction is a curious criterion for developmentalists to impose on a measure of development. "Infant

mental test scores may reflect current status without predictive significance, and it seems counter-productive to deify a criterion that is
essentially nondevelopmental in character" (pp. 715-716). The frequently
noted higher predictive validity of infant tests for medically atypical
children is probably in most cases more closely related to the stability of
the particular handicap rather than to the greater sensitivity of such tests
in the evaluation of an atypical population. A persistent handicap tends
to reduce systematically the range of testable behaviors, affecting the
validity of the test results. See Kopp (1983) for a discussion of this
phenomenon.

As a general rule, the more items there are to evaluate a child's
performance at any particular age level, the more confident the user of
the test can be of obtaining a valid picture of current functioning. In
addition, adjoining age levels should be available to reflect atypical or
uneven development, and test users are advised to remain well within the
age range specified for a particular test in order to avoid floor or ceiling
effects. On the other hand, of course, if a test is too lengthy it may be
overly tiring for the child.

Another factor to consider is the breadth of information the test
results convey. Gesell (1925) was the first to caution that "a single
summative numerical value cannot do justice to the complexity and
variability of infant development." More information can be gained
from a profile of separate subscale scores that refer to individual
behavior categories. Such differentiation is especially useful when the
purpose of the assessment is intervention planning. On the other hand,
subscale scores tend to be less reliable than summary scores since they
are based on a much smaller number of items (Sattler, 1974).

The Stanford-Binet is an example of a test that, although designed for
individuals from the age of 2, has considerable problems in these
respects when used to assess very young children. It offers only six items
at each age level six months apart—that is, at 2, 2½, 3, . . . years—and
yields a single score of mental age or deviation IQ. In an attempt to
extract more specific information, Sattler (1974) classified responses
according to their function into a profile, the so-called Binetgram.
However, the Binetgram serves to underline the test's weakness
regarding the early years. Of the seven suggested categories, only two or
three apply for children between 2 and 3½ at any given age level, and
even within categories there is little consistency. For example, the
language category is represented with three items at age 2, with four
items at 2½, with only one item at 3, and not at all at 3½ years, a time
when language development is most salient.

While a representative sampling of age-appropriate behaviors and an informative scoring system are important considerations when choosing an assessment device, another critical factor is the representativeness of the population sample on which it was standardized. The smaller and the more homogeneous the normative sample, the more cautious test users have to be when interpreting scores. This is especially true when the infant does not closely resemble the standardization group, as in the case of handicapped or otherwise atypical children. It may be advisable in such cases either to look for tests that were designed for a particular population, such as Down's syndrome (Chen & Wolley, 1978) or blind children (Reynell & Zinkin, 1975), or to adopt alternative assessment procedures to trace development, such as through symbolic play (Nicolich, 1977), or infant recognition memory (Fagan & McGrath, 1981; Zelazo, 1982), or even to correct the infant's age to make the age norms of a test more suitable, as in the case of preterm infants (Kopp, 1983).

Moreover, older tests that have not been restandardized may have less validity because they do not account for changes affecting the whole population of infants, such as general changes in perinatal care, in nutrition, in the awareness of parents regarding infant stimulation, or in the use of language. Similarly, problems may arise when tests are used transculturally (Smith, 1974).

To add to the confusion, test developers do not always agree on the age placement of particular behaviors, even within the same culture. A case in point are the mirror test items, where the behavior "smiles at image" is described as typical for 5 months by Gesell and Bayley, whereas in the Cattell and Griffiths scale it occurs among 7-month and 10-month items respectively (Brooks & Weinraub, 1976).

Finally, the test user should be aware that relatively few infant tests conform strictly to the Standards for Educational and Psychological Tests. In a 1979 survey of 78 infant tests fewer than one-third of them were found to be standardized, and fewer than one-third were found to provide any information on reliability and validity. It was also reported that in the majority of instruments administration and scoring procedures were left for the user to figure out (Johnson & Kopp, 1980). While the failure to meet test standards does not necessarily render a measure useless, the authors of the survey point out that it does place a sizable burden on the potential interpreter of the test.

With these sobering considerations in mind, let us now review some instruments frequently used with infants. We will divide them into general developmental tests and more specialized instruments designed for neonatal, temperament, language, and neuropsychological assessments. We will also describe some instruments designed to evaluate the infant's caretaking environment. Having alerted the reader to some of the problems relating to a test's reliability and validity, we have kept the respective numerical information to a minimum. On the other hand, we have thought it useful to include in our descriptions wherever possible the number of items a given test offers and the type of scores it yields, together with some information on the standardization sample.

DEVELOPMENTAL TESTS

Developmental tests are by far the largest category among infant tests. They encompass different age ranges from birth onward and their character changes with the unfolding behavioral and verbal repertoire of the child. In the following section we will introduce the Bayley as the most respected and well-researched comprehensive developmental test to date, and give an example each of short screening devices and tests based on Piaget's concepts of development. For information on other tests in the developmental category see Table 5.2.

Bayley Scales of Infant Development

This test assesses the developmental status of infants from 1 to 30 months (Bayley, 1969). It consists of three separate scales. The Mental Scale evaluates sensory-perceptual abilities, object constancy, memory, problem-solving, verbal ability, and precursors of abstract thinking. The Motor Scale assesses gross and fine motor behaviors. The Infant Behavior Record, which is completed by the examiner after the administration of mental and motor scales, rates the infants on such characteristics as social responsiveness, interests, emotions, energy level, and goal directedness as displayed during testing. Items are scored as *pass* or *fail*.

The results are expressed in terms of a Mental Development Index (MDI) and a Psychomotor Development Index (PDI). There is a total of 274 items normed at one-half-month intervals up to 5 months and at one-month intervals from 6 to 30 months. The test takes 45 to 90 minutes to complete. It was standardized on a stratified sample of 1262 children. Reliability and validity data are available.

TABLE 5.2

Other Developmental Tests

Test	Age Range	Total Items/Items for 0-3 Years / Content Area	Scoring	Total/0-3 Years Standardization Sample
Alpern-Boll Developmental Profile II (Alpern et al., 1980)	0-9 years	186/87 items / Physical, communication, academic, self-help, social	5 subscales, developmental age	3008/800 normal children stratified
Birth to Three Developmental Scale (Bangs & Dodson, 1979)	0-3 years	85/85 items / Language (comprehension and expression), problem solving, social/personal, motor	5 subscales, DQ/developmental age	357 normal children
Brisance Diagnostic Inventory of Early Development (Brisance, 1978)	0-7 years	705/569 items / Gross/fine motor, self-help, prespeech, language, general knowledge and comprehension, school-related abilities	developmental ages for all scales and subscales	not reported
Cattell Infant Intelligence Scale (Cattell, 1940)	2-30 months	95/95 items / Motor, language, adaptive, personal/social	mental age	274 normal middle-class infants, not restandardized
Gesell Developmental Schedules (Knobloch & Pasamanick, 1974)	0-3 years	374 items / Motor language, adaptive, personal/social	4 subscales developmental quotient	several small unrepresentative samples
Griffiths Mental Developmental Scale (Griffiths, 1954)	0-24 months	260/260 items / Locomotor, eye/hand, hearing, speech, performance, personal/social	5 subscales IQ/developmental age	604 normal infants in London (Engl.)
McCarthy Scales of Children's Abilities (McCarthy, 1972)	2½-8½ years	143/? items / Verbal, perceptual performance, quantitative, memory, motor, general cognitive	5 ability scales, general cognitive index	1,032/206 representative children, including mentally retarded
Vineland Adaptive Behavior Scale (Sparrow et al., 1984)	0-adult	261/? items (Survey Form) 541/? (Expanded Form) / Communication, daily living skills, socialization, motor skills	4 domain scores, 1 composite score	3,000 normal individuals, stratified, and atypical groups

The Infant Behavior Record contains 30 items that are rated on a nine-point scale. It was standardized on 791 infants of heterogeneous background.

The result of over 40 years of developmental research, this test has been praised as a "truly excellent" instrument for evaluating current developmental functioning (Damarin, 1978). Although normed on normal children up to 30 months, it has also been found useful for assessing severely handicapped children beyond that age range as long as normative tables are not used to determine scores and results are interpreted cautiously (Gerken, 1983).

The Denver Developmental Screening Test

This test (Frankenburg & Dodds, 1970) was designed to identify children with serious developmental delay from birth to 6 years. It assesses gross motor, fine motor/adaptive, language, and personal-social abilities. Of its 105 items, 75 are appropriate for children up to 3 years. Items are scored as *pass*, *fail*, *refused*, or *no opportunity*. A child of any given age will usually be tested on about 20 items. Both direct observation and maternal report are used, and results are expressed in a single score. A child who succeeds on all items is classified as normal, one failure in any one subject area is termed as questionable, and two or more failures in at least one subject area are classified as abnormal. The test takes about 30 minutes to administer. It was standardized on 1036 normal children between 2 weeks and 6 years, 816 of them under 3, from the Denver area. Data on test-retest and interobserver reliability and concurrent validity are available (Gerken, 1983; Werner, 1972).

This is a much-researched instrument that tends to underidentify "at risk" children under 30 months of age, but may be useful as a gross screening device for children in the 4- to 4½-year range (Werner, 1972). Werner questions the claim of the authors that after a few hours of training most adults could administer the test competently, pointing out that a screening tool is only as good as the sensitivity of its user.

Uzgiris and Hunt Ordinal Scales of Psychological Development

This is one of the few procedures based on a specific developmental theory, that of Piaget (Uzgiris & Hunt, 1975). Designed for infants from birth to 2 years, it consists of six different scales through which sensorimotor advances are assessed. Scale 1 relates to the development of visual pursuit and object permanence, Scale 2 to the child's use of means for obtaining desired environmental events, Scale 3 to imitation, divided into a vocal and a gestural subscale. Scale 4 focuses on the development of operational causality, Scale 5 on the construction of object relations in space, and Scale 6 refers to the development of schemata for relating to objects, for example, the changing role of toys. Response requirements vary between manipulation of objects by the infant and interactions with the examiner. The eliciting situations within each scale are arranged in hierarchical order from simple to complex.

Five different developmental stages are identified, around the ages of 0 to 3, 4 to 7, 8 to 11, 12 to 17, and 18 to 24 months. The test consists of 63 items.

The standardization sample leaves much to be desired. Two groups of 65 and 84 infants from middle-class urban families were selected to test the scales. Mean ages for achievement on each of the scales are reported as are reliability data.

NEONATAL ASSESSMENT

There are two types of neonatal tests available. One includes screening instruments that are designed to differentiate between normal and abnormal conditions in newborns. The other focuses more specifically on individual differences between newborn infants. Both have in common that they aim not for the infant's average, modal performance, but for his or her best possible performance. This sets them apart from regular developmental tests where the examiner tries to see how the child usually functions (Brazelton, 1975; Prechtl, 1982). Here we will describe only the Brazelton as an example of the second type of tests. For neonatal screening tests the reader is referred to Table 5.3.

Neonatal Behavioral Assessment Scale

This is the most comprehensive technique available today for the assessment of the behavioral and neurological status of infants from 2

TABLE 5.3
Other Neonatal Tests

Test	Age Range	Content Area	Scoring	Standardization Sample
Neurological Examination of the Full-Term Newborn Infant (Prechtl & Beintema, 1964)	1-9 days	States, posture, motility, respiration, neurological assessment		1,500 infants with history of obstetrical complications
Rosenblith Revision of the Graham Behavior Test for Neonates (Rosenblith, 1974)	1-14 days	Maturational level (motor, tactile-adaptive), sensory response (auditory, vision), irritability, muscle tension	6 subscales, general maturation index	176 normal and 81 abnormal infants (Graham's original sample)

days to 6 weeks, with special emphasis on interactive behaviors (Brazelton, 1973). It consists of a series of 20 elicited reflexes and movements rated on a four-point scale for low, medium, or high intensity of response, or absence of response, and 27 ratings of overall organization, interactive and motoric capacities, and organizational capacities relating to state control and to physiological responses to stress. Each item is administered during the appropriate behavioral stage. A nine-point rating scale is used for the behavioral items with 5 denoting expected behaviors. In addition, the newborn's overall organization is rated along the global dimension of attractiveness defined as responsiveness and contribution to interaction. Also assessed is his or her need for stimulation in order to organize his or her own responses. The NBAS takes 20 to 30 minutes to administer and 10 to 15 minutes to score. There is no single behavior quotient or numerical index. The information of interest is the pattern of behavior clusters for making a judgment of "at risk" or "normal."

The test should be administered only by a specially trained professional who has extensive experience with newborns. To ensure that examiners keep consistently high standards in scoring, they are advised to test a "normal control" as every fifth patient.

The NBAS was standardized on a sample of 54 healthy full-term white newborns in Boston. Reliability and validity studies indicate that the characteristics tapped by this scale are fairly stable (Als, Tronick, Lester, & Brazelton, 1979; Self & Horowitz, 1979).

One of the most promising uses of the NBAS has been found to be as a teaching tool for parents as well as nurses, acquainting them with the particular needs, characteristics, and abilities of individual newborns and thus helping them to provide more responsive care and to establish a more mutually satisfying relationship with the infant. This procedure has been adapted for use with premature infants (Als, Lester, Tronick, & Brazelton, 1982).

INFANT TEMPERAMENT

This is a comparatively new dimension of behavior that focuses on individual differences apart from developmental status. In a review of 26 temperament measures Hubert, Wachs, Peters, and Gandour (1982) note that in general their short-term test-retest reliability is only moderate and that levels of interparent and parent-observer agreement are low. The best known of these scales is Carey and McDevitt's Revised Infant Temperament Questionnaire.

Revised Infant Temperament Questionnaire

This is a screening device for difficult temperament in infants between 4 and 8 months (Carey & McDevitt, 1978). It consists of 95 behavioral items rated by the parents according to frequency on a six-point scale in addition to nine global temperament ratings. There are nine categories, which include activity, rhythmicity, approach, adaptability, intensity, mood, persistence, distractability, and threshold. Infants are classified as either difficult (arrhythmic, withdrawing, low adaptable, intense, negative), easy (rhythmic, approaching, adaptable, relaxed, and the like), slow to warm up (inactive, mild, negative, and so on), or intermediate. The questionnaire was standardized on 203 infants between 4 and 8 months from mostly middle- and upper-middle-class families.

LANGUAGE ASSESSMENT

Whereas the traditional emphasis in language assessment has been on articulation and phonology, as well as language structure and content, there is a growing awareness now of the pragmatic demands of language that vary with both context and function. Consequently there was a shift in the late 1970s and early 1980s away from the reliance on standardized testing in favor of descriptive, more informal assessment strategies. For an up-to-date discussion see Bryen and Gallagher (1983). The language development of very young children, because of its great variability, is even less well served by standardized testing and should only be evaluated informally, within the context of a comprehensive developmental assessment. See Table 5.4 for a selection of commonly used early language tests.

NEUROPSYCHOLOGICAL ASSESSMENT

Little is known about the usefulness of standardized tests in the assessment of infants with known or suspected brain damage. However, since certain tests are designed to assess functions thought to be located in specific areas of the brain, they may possibly help support or refute diagnostic hypotheses arrived at through an informal assessment. Hartlage and Telzrow (1983) have selected some tests they believe to tap differential functioning of the frontal, temporal, and parietal lobes of both the left and right hemispheres. They propose the following battery of tests for children between 2 and 3 years of age: Frontal lobe left hemispheric functioning is assessed through the Expressive One-Word Picture Vocabulary Test (Gardner, 1979) and right hemispheric functioning through the Developmental Test of Visual-Motor Integration (Beery; 1967). Temporal lobe left hemispheric functioning is assessed with Verbal Memory I and II, and right hemispheric functioning through the Tapping Sequence, all from the McCarthy Scales (McCarthy, 1972). Parietal lobe left hemispheric functioning is assessed with the Peabody Picture Vocabulary Test (Dunn, 1965; Dunn & Dunn, 1981), and right hemispheric functioning with Block Building and Puzzle

TABLE 5.4
Language Tests

| Test | Age Range | Total Items | | Total/0-3 Years |
		Content Area	Scoring	Standardization Sample
Developmental Sentence Analysis (Lee, 1974)	2-7 years	100 items Expressive syntax in spontaneous speech	sentence scores	200/80 normal middle-class children
Expressive One-Word Picture Vocabulary Test (Gardner, 1979)	2-12 years	110 items Sound discrimination, auditory memory, auditory processing, audiovisual association, fluency in English as second language		1,607 representative children in metropolitan area
Illinois Test of Psycholinguistic Abilities (Kirk et al., 1968)	2-7 years	345 items Auditory reception, visual reception, visual and auditory memory, visual association and closure, verbal expression, grammatic closure, manual expression, auditory closure, sound blending	12 subtest scores and developmental ages, summary score	not reported in manual
Preschool Language Scale (Zimmermann et al., 1960)	1½-7 years	103 items Auditory comprehension, verbal ability, articulation	2 subscale scores, summary score	not reported in manual
Receptive-Expressive Emerging Language Scale (Bzoch & League, 1971)	0-36 months	Language-related behavior, expressive, receptive	2 subscale scores	50 linguistically competent infants
Reynell Developmental Language Scales, Revised (Reynell, 1977)	1-5 years	177 items Expressive language, verbal comprehension	2 age levels, 2 standard scores	over 600 normal English children 6 months to 6 years

Solving from the McCarthy Scales. For information about the individual tests see Table 5.5.

When interpreting the results Hartlage and Telzrow (1983) suggest a comparison of the intactness of the two hemispheres, that is, of standard scores on the left hemispheric measures, across all lobes, with scores on the right hemispheric tasks. Another interpretation would cut across both hemispheres for a comparison of motor, that is, frontal lobe, with sensory, that is, parietal lobe functioning (Hartlage & Telzrow, 1983). However, since none of the tests or subscales of tests used in this battery was standardized on atypical populations, and they were not designed to identify neuropathology, this procedure is of questionable validity and should be considered experimental. This type of neuropsychological assessment may be too simplistic. It has been argued that the functions thought to be tapped by tests such as the above are "brain-related" but not "brain-localized," that is, that there is no simple relationship between brain and behavior. To make inferences about the damage or intactness of an infant's brain from his or her test behavior, it is necessary to make use of both new multivariate statistical procedures and clinical observations of strengths and problem-solving strategies (Dennis, 1984; Messick, 1983).

THE CARETAKING ENVIRONMENT

Here we want to present two interesting recent instruments, one focusing on the parents' perspective of their situation, the other evaluating the infant's home environment.

Parenting Stress Index

This is a self-report instrument that is designed to identify stress in parent and child systems and the related risk of deviant development in the child or of dysfunctional parenting (Burke & Abidin, 1978). There are 101 items representing the three domains of child, parent, and situational characteristics. Child characteristics include adaptability,

TABLE 5.5
Neuropsychological Test Battery

Test	Age Range	Total Items/0-3 Years Content Area	Scoring	Total/0-3 Years Standardization Sample
Developmental Test of Visual-Motor Integration (Beery, 1967)	2-8 years	15/3 items Copying form items	age equivalent	? /20 children
Expressive One-Word Picture Vocabulary Test (Gardner, 1979)		(see language tests)		
McCarthy Scales of Children's Abilities (McCarthy, 1972)		(see developmental tests)		
Peabody Picture Vocabulary Test (Dunn & Dunn, 1981; Dunn, 1965)	2½-18 years	175/9 items receptive vocabulary of Standard English	standard score	1,066/68 stratified children and adolescents

SOURCE: Hartlage and Telzron (1983).

acceptability, demandingness, moodiness, distractability, and the ability to reinforce mother. Parental characteristics include depression, attachment to the child, role restriction, sense of competence, social isolation, self-blame, marital relationships, and health. Situational characteristics include demographic factors and life events. Results are expressed as domain scores as well as a total score. The normative sample consisted of the mothers of 534 children between 1 month and 10 years with 60% under 3 years. Mothers with a fifth-grade reading level are said to complete this questionnaire in about 25 minutes.

Reliability and validity data are available and suggest that this instrument is useful not only as a screening device but as a guide to intervention and treatment planning and as a measure of the effectiveness of intervention aimed at reducing stress through brief parent consultations.

Home Observations for Measurement of the Environment—HOME

This test was designed to evaluate the home environment of children from 0 to 3 and from 3 to 6 years of age (Caldwell, 1979). The 0 to 3 scale consists of 45 items encompassing six areas:

(1) maternal warmth and emotional and verbal responsivity,
(2) avoidance of restriction and punishment,
(3) organization of the physical and temporal environment,
(4) provision of appropriate play materials,
(5) maternal involvement with the child, and
(6) opportunity for variety in daily stimulation.

The test takes a trained observer about 60 minutes to administer. Thirty items are scored during direct observation of approximately 30 minutes' duration, another 15 items form the basis of an interview with the mother. The standardization sample consisted of 174 infants from predominantly black, low SES families. There is some evidence that scores on this measure predict later cognitive performance. However, this scale is probably unsuitable for middle- and upper-class families with their more uniform standards of child rearing. A shorter version, the HOME Screening Questionnaire (HSQ) with 32 questions for the 0 to 3 age group is available (Coons, Frankenburg, Garrett, Headley, & Fandal, 1978).

SUMMARY

In summary, a great variety of tests are available to assess different areas of functioning in infants. Since very young children are notoriously variable in their behavior as well as in their rate of development, test results have to be interpreted with great caution, as estimates of current status rather than predictors of future development. Tests have a useful contribution to make if they are viewed as steps in a data collection procedure; they should never be taken as endpoints or the sum total of the identification or diagnostic process (Kopp, 1983).

In recent years new dimensions of behavior have been explored that help shape the interaction between the infant and his or her caretaking environment. Some of these dimensions can now be assessed with standardized tests and have added to the sophistication of the assessment process. Nevertheless, regardless of how well-constructed and researched they are, tests alone cannot provide the answer. As Messick (1983) points out, a valid assessment of developmental change requires a systems perspective that takes into account the host of variables involved in the child's interactions with his or her environment. For such an approach a multitude of techniques, including tests, is needed to obtain the relevant information.

6

PERVASIVE DEVELOPMENTAL DISORDERS

There has been an understandable hesitation to label infants as psychiatrically disturbed. In fact, until the most recent edition of the *Diagnostic and Statistical Manual of Mental Disorders* (DSM-III) which was published in 1980, there were no recognized psychiatric entities pertaining to infants. DSM-III cites two conditions specific for this age group: Pervasive Developmental Disorders and Reactive Attachment Disorders. This clearly signifies a big step toward the recognition of the special psychiatric needs of infants. However, it is only a beginning. As the reader may have recognized already, the problems infants can present to the world around them are multifaceted and complex and can clearly not be subsumed under two diagnostic headings. For this reason, we will discuss, in the following two chapters, the disorders referred to in DSM-III in some detail but will also outline other psychiatric conditions that can be diagnosed during the first three years of life with sufficient specificity. For each condition we will provide a brief historical note, give a clinical description, include epidemiological data if available, discuss the etiology and prognosis, and finally outline its treatment and possible prevention. Case examples will also be provided.

Pervasive developmental disorders are characterized by severe disturbances in a child's social, cognitive, language, and emotional development. These disturbances can become evident within the first 30 months of life and are not simply a reflection of delayed intellectual development, but indicate a pervasive distortion of development.

Pervasive developmental disorders, as outlined in the 1980 version of DSM-III, contain three distinct conditions: (1) Infantile Autism, (2) Childhood-Onset Pervasive Developmental Disorder, and (3) Atypical

Pervasive Developmental Disorder. Since the second condition was seen as a different illness by some clinicians and its definition had caused a great deal of controversy, a group of experts has recently met to revise DSM-III. While these revisions are not yet officially accepted, the present chapter will be based on definitions devised by this body.

The new diagnostic category will be called "Autistic Disorder" and would be subdivided into (1) Infantile Onset (before age 36 months), (2) Childhood Onset, (3) Onset Unknown, and (4) Atypical Autistic Disorder.

AUTISTIC DISORDER, INFANTILE ONSET (299.0)

Historical Note

The symptoms of early onset autism have been recognized for some 80 years. They were initially thought to be an early form of Kraepelin's Dementia Praecox and were called "dementia praecoccissima" by de Sanctis (1925). They were also seen as precursors of adult schizophrenia and hence were given the name "childhood psychoses" (Potter, 1933).

However, in 1944, Kanner described 11 children who suffered from a number of specific disturbances and called them "autistic." The main trouble these children showed was an inability to relate to others and to show appropriate interpersonal responses. Thus Kanner's patients barely seemed to notice anyone in their vicinity and exhibited stereotyped, aloof behaviors that showed few variations. On the other hand, these children also seemed to require an unchanging environment as they became anxious and acutely disturbed following the most minute changes in their surroundings. Their language development was remarkable in many ways. The children would repeat the same syllables or parts of words for long periods (called "echolalia"), never seemed to learn to use personal pronouns, and would not use speech to communicate. Kanner believed that some areas of development, such as rote memory skills, were less affected by the condition than other language skills and that the children were not generally mentally retarded (Kanner, 1944). When follow-up studies traced the development of these children into adulthood (Eisenberg & Kanner, 1956; Rutter, Greenfield, & Lockyer, 1967), it became clear, however, that some of Kanner's concepts had to be modified. For example, follow-up data documented that many autistic children were also mentally retarded (deMyer et al., 1974; Wing & Gould, 1979) and had other medical problems such as rubella (Chess, Fernandez, & Korn, 1974). The great majority of autistic children also did not end up being schizophrenic, causing the committee revising earlier editions of the *Diagnostic and Statistical Manual of Mental Disorders* to label the condition a Pervasive Developmental Disorder.

Clinical Description

The criteria for early onset autism as stated in the revised version of DSM-III are as follows:

(A) Onset before 36 months of age;
(B) A qualitative impairment in reciprocal social interactions as manifested by at least four of the following:
    (1) Failure to use eye-to-eye gaze, body posture, and gestures to moderate social interaction.
    (2) Rarely, if ever, initiates interaction play with others.
    (3) Rarely, if ever, seeks others for comfort or affection except in a mechanical way.
    (4) Rarely, if ever, offers comfort to others.
    (5) Rarely, if ever, greets others.
    (6) No peer relationships despite ample opportunities.
    (7) Rarely, if ever, imitates other people's behavior.
(C) A qualitative impairment in communication is manifested by either item 1 or at least three of the following:
    (1) No spoken language, and a failure to compensate by using alternative modes of communication such as gesture and mime.
    (2) Failure to respond to the communication of others.
    (3) If speech is present, neither initiates nor can sustain a conversation with others.
    (4) Stereotypical and repetitive use of language.
    (5) Use of "you" when they want to express "I."
    (6) Idiosyncratic use of words and phrases.
    (7) Abnormalities in pitch, stress, rhythm, and intonation of speech.
(D) A restrictive, repetitive repertoire of behaviors as manifested by at least one of the following:
    (1) A lack of varied, spontaneous "make believe" play, such as not playing house, doctor, or cowboys and Indians.

    (2) Attachment to unusual objects.
    (3) Ritualistic activities.
    (4) Stereotyped and repetitive motor mannerisms.
    (5) Preoccupation with part objects or nonfunctional elements of play
         materials.
    (6) Becomes very upset when changes are made in small details of
         environment.
  (E) Characteristics in B, C, and D may vary over time and from situation to
       situation, but are never absent.

Retrospective reports of parents suggest that autistic infants show severe delays or abnormal forms in their emotional, social, motor, and cognitive development during the first six to twelve months of life (Ornitz, Guthrie, & Farley, 1977). A minority of parents, however, maintain that their infants developed normally up to 14 or 18 months; that is, they allegedly learned a few words that they used appropriately and then within a short period lost their speech. These children are also described as having been attached to specific adults around them.

Parents often report that their infants either never showed a social smile or greeting or suddenly lost it between 12 and 18 months. They also say that their infants did not seem to anticipate being held, would not snuggle up when carried around, and in general appeared uninterested in their parents. They would also not look or smile when approached by others. However, caretakers rarely seek help until the child is about 2 years old and has failed to develop any language. At that time the family physician, witnessing the beginning mannerisms and stereotypic movement patterns of these infants, often wonders if the child is deaf. After the hearing has proved to be normal, a more detailed examination may reveal that the child in question either fears or seeks out particular noises, such as clanging pots or humming machines. At the same time, few autistic children are totally unaware of their environment as was reported in the past. This has been documented by Sigman and her group, among others (Sigman, Ungerer, Mundy, & Sherman, 1985). Sigman showed that autistic children in a modified Ainsworth Strange Situation Test (Ainsworth et al., 1978) showed muted but clearly recognizable behavioral responses upon their mother's departure and during the reunion episode. The prognostic significance of these variabilities in the interpersonal responsiveness of individual autistic children still needs to be ascertained.

Autistic children invariably show significant delays in their language acquisition. As they are also abnormal in their use of social communication, they often appear "unreachable" to their caretaking adults. Follow-up studies indicate that one-third of all autistic children never develop language and those who do will have developed some expressive language by age 5 (Eisenberg & Kanner, 1956).

When speech does develop, it is unusual in its syntax and use. Thus autistic children will not use symbolic language (for instance, they will not tell someone how they feel in comparison with someone else) and show no gestures highlighting the feelings they want to communicate. As mentioned previously, they often simply repeat what someone else has said to them (echolalia), they reverse pronouns and use big chunks of language in an effectively inappropriate fashion (for example, a child named Martha may greet a visitor by saying "How are you John? Very well, thank you, how are you Martha?"). Such speech in some way resembles a computer print-out and is devoid of affect and personal communication. This makes it distinctly different from the speech of children with developmental dysphasia or other severe linguistic disorder (Volkmar & Cohen, 1985). Autistic children's occasional use of words that have no meaning in the language of their families (called "metaphorical language") further underlines the sense of alienation and distance emanating from these youngsters.

Autistic children frequently show bizarre habits. They will look into strong lights or even the sun without blinking, may "whirl" aimlessly when turned round once by the examiner, may show strange mouthing movements and/or move part of their limbs in stereotypic fashion. Their gait and movements may seem awkward, lacking the normal smooth flow of muscle activity. They also often appear to have adopted a specific toy or object as their sole companion and vigorously resist any attempt to separate them from it. Such objects can be specific pieces of clothing like an old hat, but may also consist of toys, household utensils (a piece of rope, a pan) or a fixed item (keyholes, a lock mechanism of a door, and so on). They may also be preoccupied with sniffing or the repetitive feeling of texture of materials or want to continuously spin the wheels of toy cars. However, it is the disturbance of all spheres of development that brings about the unusual responses in these children and makes caretakers so often feel left out and rejected.

Epidemiology

Infantile autism is extremely rare, varying in different surveys from 1 in 30 to 1 in 5000 infants (deMyer, Hingtgen, & Jackson, 1981). Boys are more frequently affected with a ratio of 3 or 4 to 1 (Wing, 1981), but girls often show more severe manifestations. Autistic children are born to parents of all socioeconomic classes (Schopler, Andrews, & Strupp, 1979) and the prevalence in siblings of children with the disorder is up to 50 times more common (Greenspan, 1981). Folstein and Rutter who studied 21 same-sexed twin pairs with at least one of the children being autistic (Folstein & Rutter, 1977) presented similar data.

Etiology

The etiology of pervasive developmental disorders is unknown. Historically, one group of clinicians thought the cognitive and emotional problems of these children as secondary to the child's social deficits, which in turn were allegedly due to the child's experience of poor parenting (Bettelheim, 1967). Thus Bettelheim suggested that autistic children generally have cold and impersonal caretakers. Research has failed to support this view as it has shown parents of autistic children to have no more psychopathology than do parents of children with obvious organic disorders (McAdoo & deMyer, 1978). Other theorists suggested that autistic children failed to learn from the environment because they are excessively fearful and therefore cannot involve themselves in learning (Tinbergen & Tinbergen, 1976). More recent work by McHale, Simeonsson, Marcus, and Olley (1980) as well as Clarke and Rutter (1981) showed social communication in autistic children to increase when social demands are made on them. These findings as well as the high incidence of mental retardation suggest that these children suffer from a primary organic dysfunction.

Many authors have tried to document specific patterns of cerebral dysfunction or a specific biochemical marker in these children (Ritvo, Ornitz, Walter, & Hanley, 1970; Young, Kavanagh, Anderson, Shaywitz, & Cohen, 1982). Such a biological correlation with the psychiatric symptomatology seemed indicated especially after autistic syndromes had been observed following congenital rubella and phenylketonuria (Chess, 1971; Chess et al., 1974). However, no reliable results have been obtained although there is increasing evidence that the autistic syndrome derives from a primary cognitive dysfunction (Rutter, 1983), which may express itself in the particular difficulty these children have in their knowledge and appreciation of others. Thus work by Sigman and her group (Sigman et al., 1985) has suggested that autistic children are capable of self-recognition and can differentiate themselves from others. However, they do not seem to be able to develop a knowledge of others, which may in turn explain their lack of comprehension of their own feelings.

Differential Diagnosis

Children who are deaf or who have other sensory defects are most often misdiagnosed as autistic. Yet in contrast to autistic infants, deaf or retarded children retain their social awareness, initiate more social interactions, and show clearer indications of their attachment to their caretakers. The emotional or cognitive development of mentally retarded children may well be delayed but is far less distorted than that of autistic children. A thorough clinical evaluation, which may include an electroencephalogram, an audiological examination, and a search for possible specific neurological disorders mentioned above, usually provides a clear diagnosis. Rimland's diagnostic checklist and the Behavior Rating Instrument for Autistic and Atypical Children (BRIAAC), Validated by Cohen and others (1978), can be a useful addition to the clinical diagnostic process.

Prognosis

The prognosis is poor for the majority of these children. In Rutter's large series (Rutter et al., 1967) 60% of the children had an IQ of less than 35 five to fifteen years after the initial diagnosis, and 35% showed clear signs of organic brain syndromes; 59% lived in institutions and only 8% were in normal schools. More recent reviews (deMyer et al., 1981) found that 15% of autistic children can obtain gainful employment later in life and a similar number can work in a sheltered workshop. Outcome is significantly related to intellectual achievement as measured by psychometric tests, with those scoring below 50 in early childhood being least favored (Lockyer & Rutter, 1969). Even those who progress furthest remain mostly isolated from peers and dependent on their families all their lives.

Treatment

The first consideration for help must be given to the family of the autistic child. Parents of autistic children often feel profoundly rejected by their youngsters. They may also experience an acute mourning reaction for the baby they did not have once they become aware of the serious nature of their infant's condition. While the individual clinician will choose supportive measures most congenial to himself or herself, it is important to verbalize to the parents how hurt and rejected they must feel and how appropriate these feelings are. The clinician should also stress at the appropriate time that the abnormal behaviors of the child are not the fault of any family member or their child-rearing practices.

Nevertheless, it will take many interviews before family members can look at their child's condition, assess it realistically, and pursue appropriate treatment programs. The mourning process in parents of a handicapped child has been found to last one to two years (Thompson & Havelkova, 1982, p. 322) and to pass through various stages. There may be times when the family refuses to acknowledge difficulties that are obvious to the clinician or when its members are tempted to embrace some "miracle cure" to help their disturbed child. At other times a mother may simply want to cry and curse the world about her misfortune or will become excessively angry with the autistic child as she feels he or she demands too much time from her.

Specific treatments for autistic children that have been suggested over the years range from intensive psychoanalysis (Ward, 1970) to behavioral therapy and pharmacotherapy (Fish, Campbell, & Wile, 1968; Lovaas, Koegel, Simmons, & Long, 1973). While many of these treatment forms have not been adequately tested, there is no evidence that any one treatment alone will lead to a significant improvement in most children.

How then can the clinician help the child and his family? In our experience, in addition to his or her role as a reflector of parental feelings, the clinician can assist the parents in

(1) providing structure and consistency to the child's day-to-day activities, and

(2) reinforcing behaviors that suggest some purposeful content, which may help in the formation of an emotionally meaningful bond between the child and his or her family.

To achieve this, the judicious use of medication may be indicated. Haloperidol in small doses (0.1 mg per kilogram) may be especially helpful since this drug frequently decreases stereotypic behaviors (Mikkelson, 1982). However, Campbell (1976), who has written most extensively about the advantages and problems associated with pharmacotherapy in autistic children, has stressed how the tranquilized and subdued child may be appreciated by his or her family but may compromise his or her own development and learning capacities. Here again, the help obtained in one area of management may compromise other facets of a child's development, highlighting that up to now no effective pharmaceutical treatment has been identified and each treatment decision must be discussed thoroughly with the child's family.

Behavior modification programs likewise should not be started routinely for children under 3, although well-planned programs have reduced inappropriate behaviors and facilitated social interactions in older children (deMyer et al., 1981). The reason for this hesitation to use behavioral programs in young children is the intensive and sustained commitment they require, a factor that parents of very young children may not yet be ready to accept (Lovaas et al., 1973). Nevertheless, acutely disturbing symptoms of the young autistic child may well be tackled pharmacologically for brief periods and through behavior modifying practices if the family is committed to helping along in the treatment.

The other goal of treatment, the development of social behaviors of the child, can at times be assisted by having the child spend regular periods in a therapeutic nursery. Such a nursery can be a supportive structure for children and parents alike. The children are challenged socially and may well respond with improved prosocial behaviors. Parents may meet the caretakers of other handicapped youngsters and begin to discuss with them common problems and share in their search for potential solutions. Such group meetings have been found to be of immense value for parents once they have come through their initial mourning phase and are open to suggestions from others (Minde, Shosenberg, Marton, Thompson, Ripley, & Burns, 1980). At the same time, a skilled therapist may be able to see the minimal attempts of the autistic child to reach out to others and teach parents how to make use of them. The clinician can also help the parents protect the child from sudden waves of anxiety and panic or at least show them how to deal with such problems. Experienced personnel may also help the children with their motor coordination and speech development and by doing so show the parents that they are not alone in their battle for the growth of their daughter or son. The trusting relationship that may develop between the parents of these children and various therapists may in fact be the most important aspect of the overall intervention strategy.

In conclusion, therapy for the autistic child must be multimodal and family-centered. It may require a number of professionals, must be based on team work, and may have to be continued for many years. While the final outlook for the youngster in question is still guarded, parents and siblings usually experience significant relief by sharing their burden with others, including families similarly affected. The clinician's willingness to remain available to such families is generally greatly appreciated by them and often an essential part of the family's support system.

CASE EXAMPLE

Case 1

Jessica was 2½ years old when she was referred by her pediatrician for a hearing evaluation because she "did not seem to respond to any sound." When her hearing test showed normal auditory function, she was sent for a psychiatric consultation where she presented as an attractive, well-dressed little girl. Her father, a 34-year-old lawyer, had wondered for about one year about her "strange ways." He was especially concerned about her unwillingness to look at him, her inability to play with other children, and her terrible eating habits (she would eat all her food with her fingers and drink soup out of the bowl). Her mother, who was 32 years old and had worked as a primary school teacher until Jessica was born, was more upset by Jessica's inability to communicate and her obliviousness to the outside world and to herself. The most remarkable example of the latter had occurred only one month before when Jessica had accidentally closed the entrance door of their house on two of her fingers, necessitating seven stitches in a local emergency room. Although the surgery affected her fingers, Jessica at no time after the accident, nor during the surgery (which was performed without an anesthetic), showed any indication of pain or discomfort. Her mother also stressed how she seemed unable to discipline or train Jessica to obey family rules, such as helping to dress in the morning, and how she could not get her to eat with a spoon and stop her from throwing down flower pots and even ingesting dirt.

Developmentally, Jessica was born following an uneventful pregnancy. She cried briefly after her birth but has almost never done so since. As an infant her mother did not think her cuddly. On the contrary, she seemed to push her mother away quite actively from very early on and did not seem to be curious about herself; that is, she did not study her hands, but would spend hours curled up in a corner of her crib fingering part of her clothing. Jessica's motor milestones were normal: She sat up at 6 months and walked at 12 months. However, at 6 months she also began to stare into bright lights and at 18 months became aimlessly hyperactive and restless and could not be attracted to normal toys. Lately she had been carrying wooden sticks around, taken from her father's workbench, and would have a screaming fit when someone tried to take them away from her. Despite these severe problems, her mother had been able to socialize Jessica in some areas. For example, Jessica will keep her clothes on now and has also never touched the fire or a hot stove. She sleeps well and seems to have no liking for special foods. She is not toilet trained.

Both parents have tried to convince themselves that things will work out well in the end, although the mother, whose maternal uncle committed suicide at age 53 after a two-year period of depression, has always wondered whether Jessica had got some bad genes from her side of the family. Both parents also wondered about having other children and had begun to think about Jessica's future education.

On examination Jessica presented as an attractive little girl who roamed through the examining room, making occasional grunting noises. She fleetingly looked at the examiner twice in 30 minutes but actively resisted his attempt to touch or hold her. After some 10 minutes she wanted to leave the room and when prevented from doing so, screeched her disapproval in a high-pitched tone. Jessica could not be engaged in any play activity and did not have intelligible speech. When the examiner tried to engage her in some developmental tasks, however, she moved closer to her parents but did not touch or look at them.

ATYPICAL AUTISTIC DEVELOPMENTAL DISORDER (299.9)

This diagnosis, according to the DSM-III (1980, p. 92) criteria, should be "used for children with distortion in the development of multiple basic psychological functions that are involved in the development of social skills and language and cannot be classified as Infantile Autism."

This definition is too general to be of much clinical use, and the syndrome is a good example of the need for the further development of our current classification of infant disorders. For this and other reasons general instructions are being developed to give indications for "atypical" diagnoses in all child psychiatric conditions.

SUMMARY

Infantile autism is a reflection of an organic disorder the cause of which is not yet known. It presents as a distortion of all developmental parameters within the affected child. It has a poor prognosis as specific treatment is not yet available. However, some symptoms associated with autism can be helped by pharmacological and/or behavioral treatment, and supportive counseling for the families of affected children can bring significant relief to their suffering.

7

REACTIVE ATTACHMENT DISORDERS OF INFANCY

An attachment disorder is characterized by the absence or distortion of the bond normally developing between an infant and those who care for him or her. The essential features are signs of delayed or abnormal emotional development that secondarily may affect the biological growth of the child, but which are not due to a physical disorder.

Historical Note

The importance of an early nurturing environment for the adequate growth and development of young children has been known for many centuries and is documented in Chapter 1. In 1926, S. Freud brought a psychological dimension to the infant's physical helplessness. He stated that the biological helplessness of a young child burdens the parents with the responsibility for his or her well-being, but repeated ministrations assured the development of a mutual psychological attachment (Freud, 1959).

Despite this sensitive description of the needs of young children, until 40 years ago there were no detailed records of how children behaved when they were left by their parents. At that time D. Burlingham and A. Freud described observations they had made on young children who were separated from their parents during World War II and cared for by members of a nursery school Burlingham and Freud had established in England (Burlingham & Freud, 1942, 1944). These accounts give a clinically rich perspective of grieving infants and also show how some of them tried to repair the void left by their absent parents. However, it was R. Spitz who first pointed out the potential danger to life of emotional deprivation (Spitz, 1945). He initially reported that 37% of all infants placed in a foundling home in Mexico died within weeks after admission. Later, together with K. Wolf, he made the first systematic observations on about 100 infants who were cared for in an American penal institution (Spitz & Wolf, 1946). These babies were looked after by their mothers up to the age of 6 months, after which they were separated for about 3 months. Spitz describes the clinical picture of these infants, which was characterized by a gradual loss of interest in the environment, followed by poor weight gain, rocking or other stereotypic behaviors, and occasionally even death. He called this condition "anaclitic depression"(Spitz, 1946) and saw it as the direct result of these infants' lack of mothering and as a precursor of later depressive illness.

Other clinicians investigating early mother-infant separations (Bowlby et al., 1952; Prugh et al., 1953; Robertson, 1953; Robertson & Bowlby, 1952) and the response of young children to institutionalization (Provence & Lipton, 1962) have all obtained remarkably similar findings. Children of 6 months and older, when separated from their main caretakers, show a sequence of behaviors that John Bowlby labeled "protest," "despair," and "detachment." The protest phase, which may begin soon after the separation, often sees the child acutely distressed at having lost his or her mother by crying and looking eagerly toward anyone who may resemble this familiar figure. At the same time, the infant will usually refuse to be consoled by alternate caretakers. During the phase of despair, the child appears increasingly hopeless. He or she tends to be inactive and withdrawn and makes few demands on those around him or her. The phase of detachment at first seems to herald improvement as the infant now no longer rejects alternate care and seems to come to life again. However, as is so convincingly outlined by Bowlby (1969), such children will become increasingly self-centered, preoccupied with material things, and unable to relate to anyone in a meaningful fashion. Improvement thus is spurious and may cover up more serious characterological changes. One may well suggest, therefore, that children who have been deserted or neglected by their parents and who show signs of chronic despair or detachment exhibit the major characteristics of an attachment disorder.

There is one other body of literature, exemplified by the work of Bowlby on the structural theory of attachment, which can be taken as one conceptual route for our understanding of attachment disorders. Bowlby, in his recently revised volume entitled *Attachment* (Bowlby, 1982, Ch. 19) differentiates between the enduring "attachment a child may have toward a particular person and "attachment behaviors." For example, 2 ½-year-old Laura may be very attached to her father; that is, she is strongly disposed to seek proximity to or contact with him when she is anxious or ill. However, whether she will seek such contact depends on the momentary outside situation. Attachment behavior, in contrast, refers to any of various behaviors Laura may show to obtain the desired proximity with her father (for example, sitting on his lap, standing close to him, running toward him, or even just looking at him). Each of these behaviors then can either be absent or present at any one time, again depending on the circumstances. Yet only those proximity seeking behaviors that are triggered by the child's internal organizational system, her "attachment" that monitors potential internal and external dangers or stress, can be called attachment behaviors. Thus when Laura runs to visit and play with Jane or shares a toy with her, she may be physically very close to Jane but is nevertheless not exhibiting attachment behaviors.

This internal organizational system, which Bowlby calls attachment, according to Bretherton (1980) is never idle, but for normal functioning is nevertheless dependent on encouraging and helpful adults. If these are not available for sufficiently long periods, the whole inner control system may be shut off (Bowlby, 1980). This may leave the child unable to develop a meaningful attachment to anyone and may have him or her display symptoms such as those described by Spitz and Wolf. However, if the environment is at least partially responsive to the infant, his or her internal organizational system may still be functioning. Still, the behavior such an infant may show when his or her mother leaves him or her for a brief period and then returns is qualitatively different from that seen in infants with highly responsive caretakers. Ainsworth and her colleagues (1978), who have studied variation in attachment behaviors most thoroughly, have described two types of infant responses reflecting "secure" or "insecure" attachment. Securely attached infants will tolerate short absences from their mothers and upon their return greet them with open glee or delight. Insecurely attached infants, on the other hand, will behave very differently. Some of these infants explicitly avoid proximity to or interaction with their mothers after their return from a brief absence. These infants also seem to be little affected by their mothers' absence and in general show a tendency to be physically distant from their mothers. Ainsworth calls these infants the "avoidant babies." Another group of infants called "resistant babies" show apparent conflicts between a desire to be close to their mothers and a clear resistance to interacting with them during a reunion. These babies also often seem to be angry, and may hit their mothers or even hit themselves, further demonstrating their struggle between seeking proximity and running away. Such avoidant or resistant behaviors of insecurely attached children can dominate much of the caretaker-infant interaction and clinically present as precursors for an attachment disorder.

Clinical Description

The DSM-III criteria for an Attachment Disorder in Infancy, much like those for Pervasive Developmental Disorder, have recently been reevaluated. While the recommendations have not yet been accepted by the formal body of the Committee to Revise DSM-III, the suggestions reflect far more accurately the clinical manifestations of an Attachment Disorder and hence will be used here in modified form. The criteria are:

(A) Age of onset before 5 years,
(B) Inadequate or disturbed social relatedness in most contexts, as evidenced by at least one of the following:
   (1) Lack of age-appropriate interest to initiate or respond to most social interactions.
   (2) Fearfulness and/or hypervigilance that does not respond to comforting by caregivers.
   (3) Indiscriminate sociability (e.g., excessive familiarity with relative strangers through inappropriate requests and displays of affection).
(C) Not due to a physical disorder, mental retardation, or infantile autism.

The initial version of DSM-III requires that infants with an attachment disorder show their symptoms before they are 8 months old. However, in the present version this age range has been extended. This is based on the work of Ainsworth and associates (1978), Main and Weston (1981), and Water and associates (1979), all of whom have documented the persistence of manifestations of insecure attachments far beyond the age of 12 months.

The lack of the infant's age-appropriate interest in a primary caretaker should not suggest a specific source of this deficit, although the revised DSM-III manual states there is a presumption that grossly inadequate care is responsible for the disturbed behavior of the infant. In fact, in the suggested new outline an attachment disorder can also be diagnosed when the infant has experienced psychological or physical abuse and neglect, or a repeated change of primary caregivers, making it impossible for stable attachments to occur.

It is obvious to the clinician that the lack of care or sensitivity as well as active physical abuse can be important precursors for a deviant or faulty development of the attachment system within a child. On the other hand, some children for reasons beyond their parents' control may be very difficult to look after and present with signs of neglect despite serious attempts by their parents to care for them. Case number 2, presented in detail later, is an example. Here a twin infant who, because of premature birth, had to remain in hospital for a number of months was further handicapped by a tracheotomy at 6 months. While his twin brother spent this time with his mother at home, Ben, who because of his operation could neither cry nor show his wishes, had to remain in hospital. His mother, who had her hands full with his twin brother James and her two other children, could visit Ben only sporadically. While the professional staff of the hospital tried hard to stimulate Ben, he weighed only 8 pounds at 3 months corrected age, and was a scrawny, unhappy, and irritable little boy.

In addition to the difficulties children may present for their care-takers, it has also been shown that attachment behavior can be quite person-specific. In studies of physically abused infants Gaensbauer and Sands (1979) and Gaensbauer and Harmon (1982) have documented that infants aged 12 to 21 months who had been abused by their fathers showed very abnormal fear responses and/or the lack of other behaviors usually associated with attachment toward other males but appeared much less disturbed in the company of women. This as well as other work (see, for example, Blehar, 1974), underlines the complexity of attachment reactions and the danger of simplifying the etiology of disturbances in their development.

The signs of the infant's disordered emotional development are outlined by the criteria mentioned in the above description and need little further elaboration here. However, it may be important to stress that a lack of reciprocity implies the infant is unwilling or unable to engage with another person using any one of his or her basic sensory organs. For example, such infants may not engage in mutual looking with the caretaker, may not babble in response to him or her, and may not play any give-and-take games. As such interactive processes are very basic building blocks of an infant's day-to-day development, disturbances in this area must be taken seriously.

Children who will not engage in social interactions and who also show poor weight gain are seen as suffering from the "failure to thrive" syndrome. This syndrome, which is characterized by weight and growth below the tenth percentile following an *initially normal* growth and weight and an absence of organic disease, is commonly found in neglected or institutionalized children. However, serious parental insensitivity to an infant's needs, abrupt weaning, or general tension between parents can also be expressed by the infant's refusal to eat. A more detailed discussion of eating disorders will be given in Chapter 8.

The absence of mental retardation or minor physical disorders is often difficult to ascertain as the infant may clinically appear to be retarded or may have contracted secondary physical complications. However, a good physical examination and history will usually allow proper diagnosis.

Epidemiology

There are no data available on the prevalence, sex ratio, or familial patterns of this condition. However, Call (1980, p. 2590) states that failure to thrive has been observed in as many as 1% of all infants.

Etiology

As has been mentioned before, an attachment disorder is usually the result of insufficient caretaking practices. The reasons that may make a mother or father incapable of providing the necessary psychological care for their infant are diverse and require the clinician to take a good history and make sensitive observations of all the family members during his or her intake interview. In general, however, an attachment disorder can be due to parental or infant deficiencies, although they are most commonly a reflection of difficulties in both partners.

Parental Causes

Both mental and physical disease can impede sensitive caretaking. Parents suffering from any major mental disorder, especially a depression or postpartum psychosis, may be unable to read the infant's signals for hunger or discomfort and may introduce serious distortions in the attachment process. Likewise, serious personality disorders can change parental interpretations and attributions of their infant's behavior and result in deviant behavior.

Physical diseases associated with pain and weakness requiring repeated hospitalizations of the major caretaker can equally disrupt the attachment process and lead to serious disorders in the infant. Parental diseases in turn can be acute or chronic and may vary in duration and severity.

The early history of the primary caretaker may also give important clues, as we know now that the ability to look after an infant is significantly related to one's own upbringing (Frommer & O'Shea, 1973; Wolkind, 1977). Poverty, early emotional and physical abuse, and other conditions associated with poor self-esteem are therefore often found in parents of infants with attachment disorders.

Infant Causes

Children who have been born prematurely or with specific malformations (e.g., phocomelia or severe facial abnormalities) are often extremely difficult to look after. Parents may also need to mourn the loss of their wished-for child and may become emotionally unavailable to such an infant for some time (Wolkind et al., 1984). Colicky and poorly regulated or crying infants likewise are hard to soothe and enjoy, which can create an interactional pattern leading to deficient attachment development.

Differential Diagnosis

Attachment disorders must be distinguished from mental retardation and autism. Children who are severely mentally retarded may not show age-appropriate social and emotional patterns. However, a thorough examination will reveal a delayed overall development. Autistic children will exhibit far more bizarre symptoms and usually have parents who are competent caretakers. Yet some autistic infants may be so difficult to "read" for a parent that neglect and consequent additional attachment problems can occur together.

Prognosis

Attachment disorders may be transient or intermittent, depending on environmental circumstances and constitutional-maturational factors. They may range from mild to severe. While mild forms may be self-limiting as children who become older can seek out relationships with adults more independently, severe forms of the disorder can lead to permanent stunting of the child's personality and in some cases even to the death of the infant. Children who are "avoidant" or "resistant" babies, that is, who show a moderately abnormal pattern of attachment behavior at 12 to 18 months, may continue to show little interest in interpersonal interactions nine months later (Main & Weston, 1981) and be less competent socially as well as less curious and sympathetic to other children's distress at 3½ years (Water et al., 1979). Arend and associates (1979) as well as Erickson and her colleagues (1985) have extended the follow-up period of such children up to the fifth and sixth year and found children who were insecurely attached in infancy to be significantly less resourceful and show less resilience; that is, they find it hard to modify their level of control according to circumstances both in school and at home.

These data, together with those of others (for example, Rutter et al., 1981; Sroufe, 1982) suggest that attachment disorders of children older than 18 months are not easily modified. As the ability to form close and intimate relationships, however, is one of the mainstays of a healthy emotional life, it follows that the prognosis of attachment disorders is potentially poor.

Treatment

The treatment of choice for attachment disorders is the improvement of the infant's care. This is best brought about after a careful and comprehensive evaluation of the child's caretakers and an assessment of the infant's strengths and vulnerabilities. Treatment criteria are (1) to refrain from adding new stresses in the form of separation or hospitalizations to the infant's life if they are not strongly indicated by external difficulties and (2) to make use of those people for treatment who are most meaningful to the caregivers. This means that the physician may be a rather peripheral member of the treatment team with public health nurses or other paramedical personnel being the essential treatment agents (Fraiberg, 1980). (3) Clinicians should aim to assist the original caretakers in their attempts to look after the infant properly. Too many clinicians initially place infants with attachment disorders in foster homes or other substitute caretaking situations instead of searching for the strengths within the biological parents and attempting to develop them.

Specific treatment may consist of pointing out sensory stimuli to which the infant may be hypersensitive and demonstrating to the parents how their child may need to be exposed to these stimuli slowly and be comforted gently. Caretakers of withdrawn and unresponsive infants may have to learn how to use novel stimuli to gradually reengage their infant (for instance, by singing to the infant or exaggerating certain facial expressions). Parents may also have to learn about baby's favorite mode of interaction (for example, does their son like being touched or having his skin rubbed? Does he like to listen to songs or prefer to hear a speaking voice?). Some parents may also require individual therapy as the pains and difficulties they experienced during their own childhood may have been reawakened by their newborn infant or toddler and make them incapable of providing for him or her. Some parents may even require proper medical treatment for themselves.

It must be stressed again that external, interpersonal, or intrapersonal problems rarely exist in isolation from each other (Greenspan, 1981) and must be tackled together by an appropriately wide system of support and rehabilitation.

CASE EXAMPLE

Case 2

Ben, aged 6 months, and his mother Mrs. C., aged 25 years, were seen in consultation because the nurses on the ward to which Ben had been admitted for the care of his tracheotomy found him to be listless and significantly delayed in his motor, adaptive, and personal social development. Thus he did not sit up nor did he want to be held. He also did not play any social games such as peek-a-boo and in general lay passively in his bed. Mrs. C. had also mentioned to the nurses that "she could not feel close to Ben" and was pleased to meet with someone who could possibly help her to overcome these indifferent feelings.

Ben was one of twins who were born at 30 weeks gestation, weighing 1020 and 1120 grams. The delivery of the babies, in contrast to that of their two older siblings 3 and 6 years ago, had been very traumatic as Mrs. C. lived in a small village some 70 miles outside a major city. After going into labor prematurely, she had been told by her general practitioner that he could not handle the expected twins in the local hospital. During the ambulance ride into town, however, labor progressed very quickly and both infants were born prior to reaching the hospital. Mrs. C. even at that moment recalled feeling closer to Ben's brother James as he was the bigger by 100 grams and cried more vigorously and in many ways seemed to be a "fighter." When James suffered a number of complications in the intensive care unit, Mrs. C. felt even closer to him and became increasingly anxious about her "lack of love" for Ben. She tried to cope with this by forcing herself to spend more time visiting Ben but found herself looking at James and thinking of him while standing at Ben's incubator.

After 2½ months both children were discharged. Mrs. C. had made sure that both infants would come home together so as not to favor one over the other. However, Ben would not take sufficient milk from her breast and had to be switched to a bottle, while James continued to nurse. Ben's weight gain, as a possible consequence, fell increasingly behind, and after 3 months at home he had only gained 2 pounds. At that time Ben contracted an apparent cold and his occasional raspy breath became much worse, requiring him to be admitted to hospital. At the hospital a diagnosis of subglottic stenosis was made. When conservative treatment failed and Ben developed a grand mal seizure, he had a tracheotomy to relieve his respiratory difficulties.

At the time of the psychiatric consultation, Ben had been in hospital for nine days and weighed 8 pounds 2 ounces. Mrs. C. had visited him almost daily, although she had always brought along James so as to "not miss a breast feed." James weighed 12 pounds 10 ounces. On examination Ben was a scrawny, anxious-looking infant who showed little interest in the examiner. While he was not formally tested it was interesting to observe that he had achieved a number of developmental milestones but made no interactional use of them and showed no apparent pleasure in them. For example, Ben could bring his hands over the mid-line (a 16-weeks item) but never in fact played with his hands or fingers. Likewise, he could lift his head and support himself on his forearms yet was not interested in doing so but slept about 18 hours a day. When observed with his mother the examiner was struck by Ben's apparent avoidance of her. Thus he would look at her quite impassively but never smile or generate any other voluntary interaction. For example, when mother tried to engage him in a verbal dialogue, Ben initially appeared to listen to her sounds but soon began to whimper as if he did not want to hear her voice any more. Ben's general developmental delay was especially worrisome to the nurses as they had made a great effort to sensitively stimulate him during the early days of his hospitalization, yet saw no change in his behavior.

Physically, Ben showed no abnormalities except for his low weight and his generally decreased muscle tone. His tracheotomy functioned well although his mother was greatly distressed by the "hole in his throat" and his inability to cry.

As both parents had experienced psychological difficulties during their early years, we felt that Ben's difficulties were related to (1) his mother's feeling of being abandoned by her local physician, which in turn awakened memories of earlier abandonment by her own parents; and (2) her disappointment and her wish to have her husband take over the total care for one infant. As Ben's father had not been willing to help her significantly with Ben and since during their marriage he had depended on her for all major decisions, which frequently enraged her, we felt that part of the "lack of love" Mrs. C. showed toward Ben was also a reflection of her angry feelings toward her husband.

As a consequence our treatment aimed to increase Mr. C.'s sense of competence by helping him to overcome a severe learning disability.

This allowed him to become somewhat more active with his wife and to support her especially in the care of the older children. Mrs. C. was also seen in individual psychotherapy to work through some of her angry feelings, and at the same time she was encouraged to look after Ben as much as possible. The thought here was to have Ben experience things with his mother and expose him to her caretaking.

While Ben remained shy and rather passive, he gradually began to show a clear preference for his mother and one particular nurse. This eventually led to a significant increase in his cognitive and emotional development and finally to his discharge home after some 3 months of hospitalization.

SUMMARY

An attachment disorder is a condition that affects an infant's development of love for his or her caretakers and the world in general. The disorder is primarily caused by a mismatch between the needs of the infant and the caretaking abilities of the parents or other primary caretakers. Treatment must aim to build or rebuild a positive relationship between the baby and those who look after him or her. This may require the help of different medical and nonmedical professionals. Failure to reestablish the attachment process at an early age may significantly compromise the ability of a child to develop positive self-esteem and social skills and to feel safe to trust others in the future.

8

EATING DISORDERS

Historical Note

In Chapter 2 we examined the significance eating has for the emotional development of the normal infant and briefly explored how psychoanalytic and other theorists viewed disorders of this function. While summarizing the opinions of different clinicians and researchers on the importance of early feeding may seem to be an unwarranted simplification of the issue, it can be said that most writers agree that the satisfactory experience associated with eating and being fed is one of the most elementary basic tasks of a newborn infant. Failure to gain pleasure and satisfaction through eating can therefore have important consequences for both the biological and psychological development of an infant. At the same time eating is one of the first criteria parents of a newborn use to validate their parenting competence, and the enduring social importance of eating or of having a meal together is clearly a reflection of the ongoing significance of this early interaction.

There are obviously a wide range of causes that may interfere with an infant's proper eating behavior. These range from primarily organic defects to mother-infant tensions that are expressed through food refusal. Yet whatever the reason for the infant's failure to eat sufficiently, parents are usually seriously affected and feel personally responsible for their infant's behavior.

Professional concern for a baby's proper food intake has had a long history. As one French physician estimated, nine out of ten infant deaths in the 1750s were due to the mismanagement of feeding (Hardyment, 1984, p. 6). Holt (1897), who in many ways was the predecessor of Dr. Spock for the North American parent in the first half of the twentieth century, was the first pediatrician to call attention to nonorganic failure to thrive and the psychological reasons for food refusal.

While the average contemporary parent is far more knowledgeable about the nutritional needs of infants, there are still a large number of infants who are taken to a physician during the first two years of life because of difficulties in this area. In fact, it has been suggested that eating or feeding disorders are "a more common cause of under-nutrition during the first year of life than deprivation or poverty" (Krieger, 1982, p. 83).

Yet among the five disturbances in eating described in the DSM-III classification, only two are relevant for infants. These are pica and rumination disorders of infancy, both rare conditions. The reasons for the discrepancy between the DSM-III and the clinical relevance of eating disorders for young children is unknown but may be related to the interactional nature of these difficulties, best expressed by the varying emphasis of some authors on eating (the infant's part) versus feeding (the caretaker's part). Since the authors of DSM-III recognized only behavioral, psychological, or biological dysfunctions (DSM-III, 1980, p. 6), there was little room for abnormal behaviors that may reflect a conflict between an individual and those around him. The problems that arise from this stand—especially in the classification of disorders of infants and young children, where difficulties are frequently reflections of interactional maladaptations—are formidable.

To bridge this gap, in the present chapter we will add one diagnostic category to the eating disorders outlined in DSM-III. After a discussion of pica and the rumination disorder of infancy we will describe the more common eating or feeding problems of infancy, which we will call "Developmental Eating Disorders of Infancy."

PICA (307.52)

Pica is the persistent eating of nonnutritive substances. Infants may eat paint, plaster, cloth, hair, or other similar substances. They do not usually show an aversion to other food.

Clinical Description

The criteria for pica as stated in DSM-III are:

(A) Repeated eating of nonnutritive substances for at least one month.

(B) Not due to another mental disorder such as infantile autism or schizophrenia or a physical disorder.

Children who present with this disorder are frequently mentally retarded. However, in a child from a large family or low socioeconomic group or where siblings do much of the caretaking, pica may be an expression of lack of social training, supervision, or lack of stimulation. In addition, there are some nonretarded children who eat nonnutritive substances in a secret fashion, almost as if they were enjoying it. These children may again come from conflicted families and will reveal specific dynamic reasons for their unusual behaviors.

There is no evidence that pica is related to an attempt by the infant to make up specific nutritional deficiencies (Krieger, 1982, p. 92). While some children with pica have been shown to suffer from iron deficiency (Gutelins et al., 1962), this may be a common result of poor parenting and not reflect a causal relationship.

Epidemiology

Pica usually begins between 12 and 14 months, although some children will show it earlier. While infants with this disorder may eat hair and cloth, older children may ingest animal droppings, cigarette butts, bugs, sand, or pebbles. Most children will put such things into their mouths at one time or another. Yet only those who are poorly supervised or who are retarded will fail to learn what to eat and what not to eat.

There is no sex preference for pica.

Differential Diagnosis

The differentiation of pica from infantile autism is fairly easy as autistic children will often show bizarre behaviors, disorders in their language, and an unwillingness to relate to others.

Treatment

This depends on the underlying problem. Neglectful parents must be appropriately supported and the infant medically examined for hair balls in the intestinal tract.

Prognosis

The condition is usually self-limiting; but some children continue to eat unsavory materials right into adolescence and adulthood, making the prognosis variable.

RUMINATION DISORDER OF INFANCY (307.53)

Clinical Description

The diagnostic criteria for this disorder as stated in DSM-III are:

(A) Repeated regurgitation without nausea or associated gastrointestinal illness for at least one month following a period of normal functioning.
(B) Weight loss.

The important criterion of this condition is the repeated regurgitation after a meal, which is followed by attempts to rechew or reswallow the regurgitated food. Some of these children, according to Krieger (1982, p. 89) are bright-eyed hyperactive infants whose parents seem to overstimulate them. Others are far more lethargic, passive infants, who appear to enjoy retasting their regurgitate and may show other signs of maternal deprivation. Krieger believes that the hyperactive group of infants are younger (less than 6 months) and have a far better prognosis than the deprived ruminators.

Most infants who regurgitate substantial amounts of food will end up vomiting some of it and be at risk for undernutrition. In fact, the nondramatic way a ruminating passive infant may gradually lose weight is often not detected and can lead to severe undernutrition and even death. A passive infant who may have a less vigilant mother is most at risk here, although one can find malnourished infants even among hyperactive and overstimulated babies. Both types of children will be hungry right after a vomited meal although refeeding may lead to renewed regurgitation.

Epidemiology

The disorder usually starts between 3 and 12 months, is equally common in boys and girls, and very rare. However, some reports claim that the mortality rate for malnutrition due to rumination disorder can reach 25% unless feeding through an indwelling duodenal catheter is instituted. Chronic malnutrition can also compromise other areas of development, causing discouragement of caretakers and further developmental delays.

Differential Diagnosis

Congenital abnormalities such as pyloric stenosis or gastrointestinal infections can cause regurgitation of food, especially if the infant also suffers from cerebral palsy or any other condition affecting muscle tone. Mental retardation must also be ruled out as here children may not be able to coordinate the various muscle groups involved in the feeding process.

Treatment

This depends on the underlying process. Overstimulated infants may have to be propped up after feeding to help them keep their food down. Parents must be counseled either to provide their infants with age-appropriate routines or to stimulate them more actively. In some cases, medical management of the malnutrition has to take precedence as it may save the infant's life. Ruminants can be difficult to change and parents may become frustrated and alienated from the child. The clinician must be aware of these feelings and deal with them in a sensitive and appropriate fashion.

Prognosis

The long-term prognosis of rumination disorders is good as it is usually self-limiting. However, parents who become discouraged or angry with their infants and remain so even after the symptoms subside are clearly not ideal caretakers and may compromise the further growth and development of their children.

DEVELOPMENTAL EATING DISORDERS OF INFANCY

Problems of eating and feeding are of great importance in infancy because of their high frequency, nutritional implications, and psychological impact on children and their families. DSM-III does not describe a general developmental feeding disorder. The diagnostic criteria for the condition mentioned here are derived from the authors' clinical experience and must therefore be taken as an expression of their opinions.

The causes of feeding problems are extremely varied. They range from specific physical disorders such as mechanical obstructions or neuromotor dysfunctions over allergies to purely behavioral or interactional factors. As this volume deals with psychological disorders of infants, the present chapter discusses primarily those symptoms of an eating disorder that are the result of psychological difficulties.

Diagnostic Criteria for Developmental Eating Disorders of Infancy

(A) Active or passive refusal of food leading to an inadequate food intake as manifested by one or more of the following symptoms:
   (1) Chronic refusal to suck, swallow, or open the mouth when food is offered.
   (2) Refusal or delay in self-feeding.
   (3) Meal-time temper tantrums.
   (4) Regurgitation or vomiting of major portions of a meal within 30 minutes.
(B) Bizarre or highly unusual food habits as indicated by at least two of the following symptoms:
   (1) Chews or swallows extremely slowly, extending a meal beyond 45 minutes.
   (2) Extreme faddiness and multiple food dislikes.
   (3) Prolonged insistence on puréed or other forms of food appropriate for younger children.
(C) Duration of disturbance for at least 3 months.

(D) Onset before the age of 36 months.
(E) Not due to an organic disturbance of a mechanical, neuromuscular, or allergic nature.

Refusal of food can begin shortly after birth. The infant may not wake up for a feed, refuse to suck, or take in only small amounts during a feeding. After age 3 months an infant may actively tighten his or her lips when approached with a bottle or spoon as if to protest the caretaker's intrusion into his or her life space. At that time regurgitation or vomiting major portions of a feed also becomes more common. Infants may seem to take the bottle reasonably well but within minutes of finishing it will vomit most of it back up. After 12 months of age serious fights over food may take place as infants want to achieve a sense of independence, yet still maintain close emotional ties with their caretakers. Feeding wars may center around control of the spoon or the amount of food, and lead to dishes of food being thrown on the floor repeatedly, or food being actively spit out.

In other cases infants may refuse to participate in the feeding process. They will be uninterested in experimenting with a spoon or fork, refuse to feed themselves cookies, and in many other ways show a gross lack of interest in all matters relating to feeding.

Clinically, such an underfed infant may present as irritable and scrawny looking or as exceptionally quiet and sleepy. Mothers may describe the latter groups of infants as generally easy babies who cry little and are easily satisfied. Both breast and bottle fed babies can develop feeding problems. In fact "easy-going" breast-fed babies tend to be underfed more often than those fed by bottle as the amount of food taken in is often not known in the breast-fed group.

Excessive food faddiness is more common in children of 1 year and older. While most children will show specific food preferences during their infancy, in this condition a child refuses to eat a wide variety of foods or demands them to be prepared in specific ways. For instance, a child may eat nothing but pudding or will touch nothing that looks green or red.

Feeding problems of less than three-months' duration may be related to transient stresses in the life of the infant. For example, a change in babysitters, a maternal illness, or the birth of a sibling may all affect the appetite or faddiness of a toddler. Infections or other physical illnesses of the infant will also frequently decrease his or her food intake as will the introduction of new foods.

Epidemiology

There are few reliable data on the incidence, sex ratio, or familial patterns of this condition. However, Jenkins and associates (1980) in a study examining the symptomatology of all 359 infants aged 6 to 36 months in a London borough, found 6% of the mothers to report significant problems in feeding their infants and 12% to report food fads as early as 6 months after birth. This remained virtually the same at 1 year but went up to 24% (poor and slow to feed) and 15% (food fads) at 18 months. At 36 months 34% of all infants ate poorly and 23% displayed food fads. Richman (1981), in a similar study of 3-year-old children, found 12% of her mothers to report moderate or serious feeding problems. Forsyth and associates (1984) examining some 370 infants followed by a private pediatrician in the greater New Haven area reported that at age 4 months 17% of the breast-fed and 20% of the formula-fed infants had moderate or severe problems with feeding or spitting up, while an additional 12% and 10% were described as being colicky. There were no sex differences.

Problems with food texture often begin in the later part of the first year of life. Illingworth and Lister (1964) in fact suggest that there is a sensitive period for the introduction of solid foods around 6 or 7 months. If parents failed to introduce solids then, the child, according to these authors, will be less likely to accept solid foods for some time to come.

Etiology

Eating disorders most frequently are a reflection of the caretakers' inability to understand their infant's emotional needs. This in turn may be due to well-intentioned parental actions that are nevertheless out of phase with the infant's developmental needs. For example, Palmer and associates (1975) have documented that children who are physically handicapped or who have a history of a serious physical illness frequently develop feeding problems because food fads, or other attempts to manipulate the parents through particular eating behaviors that would normally not be tolerated, are condoned by their families. On the other hand eating disorders commonly originate during the hospitalization of young children as they cannot tolerate the institutionalized way their meals are prepared and fed to them. Such eating problems are often carried over into the home and can persist for many months.

While investigators traditionally have tried to establish a relationship between specific maternal background factors such as anxiety and feeding disorders (see Carey, 1968; Ottinger & Simon, 1964), workers have also attempted to demonstrate the importance of the mother's subjective perception to her later feeding experiences. Thus Forsyth and his group (1984) found feeding difficulties to be significantly more common in families where the mother at birth had expressed concern whether she would be able to manage to "feed her infant" and where she reported older siblings to have "allergies." While the literature in this area is often impressionistic, two basic interactional patterns seem to be associated with feeding disorders. Parents who report battles during mealtimes are generally highly organized obsessional people who appear to need much control over their infant's day-to-day behaviors. Other mothers set up feeding disorders by introducing solid foods before 4 to 6 months in the belief that this will help the infant to sleep through the night. As cereals, the most commonly chosen solid food, do not have a higher caloric density than milk, sleep will not be increased by these practices. More seriously, however, there is good evidence (Krieger, 1981, p. 18) that infants under the age of 6 months are not able to express satiety and cannot yet overcome the force of the spoon. To force feed such infants, therefore, may lead to later overweight and/or battles at mealtimes.

Mothers who are generally neglectful tend to present with children who are underfed but instead of fighting seem passively to endure their deprivation. Such infants may show constitutionally weak responses to maternal overtures or fail to display strong signals of hunger or satisfaction. This, in turn, may lead to a "poor fit" (Thomas, 1981) between the parents and their infant. Parents who suffer from major psychiatric disorders such as depression or have a severely deprived personal background may likewise fail to meet their infant's nutritional needs. Such infants will often appear passive and show delays in various developmental areas.

Finally, there are a significant number of infants whose eating difficulties were initially a reflection of some biological abnormality and only secondarily become of psychological significance. Infants who are born with duodenal-esophageal fistula (an open connection between the windpipe and the esophagus) are a good example. These infants cannot take any food by mouth as all food will end up in the lungs. They are thus fed through a gastric tube that is placed directly in the stomach during a minor operation. In addition, however, they are not allowed to suck their fingers as this would increase saliva production, which, in turn, might be swallowed and lead to pneumonia. For this reason their hands are usually tied to a pillow until an operation, separating the windpipe and the esophagus, can be performed. As this may take many weeks, the whole relationship of the parents to such an infant is usually profoundly affected, and even postoperative feeding behaviors are frequently distorted and problematic. As more and more children with serious neonatal conditions or congenital abnormalities are treated today with the help of complex medical procedures, disorders of eating can be expected to be an increasingly common condition.

Differential Diagnosis

All feeding disorders must be medically evaluated as several medical conditions can lead to problems in food intake. For example, immature neonates and infants with diffuse CNS damage frequently have non-specific feeding problems. Children with malignancies that are treated with cytostatic drugs likewise frequently do not want to eat. Oto-pharyngeal dysfunctions due to movement disorders (for example, in upper motor neuron disease) or disorders associated with hypotonia (for example, chalasia) will usually lead to feeding difficulties. Specific abnormalities of the nasogastric area such as cleft lip or stenosis in the esophagus will likewise cause problems in feeding.

The second group of children who must be distinguished from those with developmental eating disorders are children with "environmental failure to thrive" (Barbero & Shaheen, 1967), also called nonorganic failure to thrive syndrome (NFTT). It is associated with growth retardation for which no organic cause can be demonstrated. Onset is usually between 3 and 12 months and about 1% of all pediatric hospital admissions show this syndrome (Hannaway, 1976). Unfortunately, there is no consensus about the etiology of the NFTT syndrome. For example, Egan and his colleagues (Egan et al., 1980) have proposed two syndromes, one of which describes infants between 8 and 18 months who become so embroiled in a struggle for autonomy with their parents through food that weight loss results. Woolston (1983) has described three subtypes of NFTT, relating to problems of attachment, caloric-protein malnutrition, and pathological food refusal. Drotar (1985) in a very extensive summary of the recent literature cites more than 250 references without arriving at a clear etiology, treatment, and outcome for the condition.

Psychological dwarfism, also called "deprivation dwarfism" (Silver & Finkelstein, 1967), in contrast to a developmental eating disorder, is also associated with developmental delays in the cognitive and emotional sphere. It has its onset between 18 and 48 months of life and in one study (Guilhaume et al., 1982) has been associated with a reversible hypopituitarism. However, there is increasing evidence that many infants with disorders of sufficient weight gain and growth have both caretakers who are overburdened and emotionally unavailable (Pollitt, 1975) as well as insufficient caloric intake.

Prognosis

The majority of children exhibiting a feeding disorder will cease to show serious eating problems after the age of 36 months. However, children who were reported by their mothers to be difficult eaters in early childhood showed a higher incidence of general behavioral problems (40% versus 15% in a controlled population) during early school age (Richman & Graham, 1982). This would imply that the struggles between a child and his or her caretakers may shift from eating to other areas of psychological functioning and that the overall outlook of the condition is more serious than had earlier been predicted (Rae-Grant et al., 1983, p. 173).

Treatment

The treatment of a developmental feeding disorder must be tailored to both the biological difficulties of the child and to the underlying problems in the parent-infant relationship. Thus, we initially want to obtain detailed information about the infant's feeding history, his or her weight, and possible organic vulnerabilities. This may include information from the infant's pediatrician or other health care professionals. If the infant shows signs of an organic problem, it is often useful to obtain the help of an occupational therapist who may assist the parent in decreasing the hypertonicity or other oral motor abnormalities (Lewis, 1982).

Once organic conditions have been excluded or are treated appropriately, it is useful to begin any psychological treatment by discussing the normal expectations of feeding patterns or stages relevant to the infant in question with his or her parents. For example, in a 6-month-old baby techniques of introducing solid foods and the respect for an infant's beginning food preferences should be brought up. In toddlers parents may need to hear that messiness is a part of feeding for an infant and premature emphasis on neatness often leads to problems in food intake.

Once this is done, one may help parents who are overanxious but show no serious personality disorder by developmental counseling as outlined by Fraiberg (1980) and Minde and Minde (1981). In families with toddlers this may be coupled with a behavioral management program for the infant. For example, a 2-year-old who refuses to eat anything that is not cut into tiny pieces may be given increasingly bigger chunks of food but left alone during a meal to deemphasize the confrontational aspects of the eating process. Any improvement in eating should be rewarded by the parents with an extra story after the meal or another activity enjoyed by the child and parent together. Food rewards (such as giving the child two puddings after eating the bread) should be avoided. It may be better to consider the child's likes and dislikes and provide a balanced diet with little or none of the hated food as children have a right to enjoy their food. Infants who are difficult to rouse and who have a more passive constitution need more frequent feeds together with more external stimulation.

As a rule, the pleasure of mealtimes can be enhanced by

(1) having meals of a predetermined length (30 minutes, for example) with foods being removed thereafter;
(2) offering no snacks between meals;
(3) have children above 12 months feed themselves for at least part of their meal;
(4) keep portions small as they can always be added to.

It should be stressed again, however, that a good number of feeding problems reflect more problematic parenting disorders. Treatment may have to be more parent centered with individual counseling of the parent exploring his or her own parenting experiences, expectations of the infant, or fears or anxieties regarding the child's future. Such treatment may also require a more carefully constructed behavioral program to provide the child with the needed calories and avoid more radical surgical interventions (such as a gastrostomy). Such programs may require the assistance of behaviorally trained individuals and should be initiated only if more supportive measures have failed.

CASE EXAMPLE

Case 3

Jennifer E. was 8 months old when her pediatrician asked for psychiatric help. The referral had been triggered by Jennifer's father threatening to leave his wife because "she spends all her time feeding Jennifer and never talks to me." Despite these intense feeding attempts by mother, Jennifer was so seriously underweight (her weight at 8 months was 10 pounds 8 ounces) that she had been hospitalized 1 week prior to the consultation. Traditional pediatric management seemed to have failed.

Jennifer was the first child of a middle-class couple in their mid-thirties. Her mother came from a very strict family, her father being a senior police officer. She had always obeyed her superiors and believed in exercising self-control. She had worked as a nurse in an operating room of a general hospital for ten years and had been in two minds about having a baby, wondering whether she was too old to be a mother or whether she and her husband could afford a baby.

Jennifer's father was born and raised in New Zealand. He had come to North America for studies but remained after he graduated, although he planned to return home "after he had made enough money." The exact time of this return had never been specified. Mr. E. worked as a computer specialist in a big firm but spent all his spare time renovating old homes, which he sold after he had finished the work. As the E. family always lived in the homes that the father renovated, the couple had moved six times since they married six years ago.

Mrs. E.'s pregnancy proceeded without complications until the 29th week when she began to go into labor. Hospitalization with strict bed rest calmed things down again but renewed contractions led to Jennifer's birth at 31 weeks, when she weighed 1380 grams. Her mother was petrified that Jennifer would die and spent all her time in the hospital. However, the little girl had a generally good postnatal course and was discharged home after six weeks weighing 2510 grams. Mother was instructed to feed her 3 ounces every three hours and return to the neonatal follow-up clinic after two weeks. Things went fairly well for three weeks, although her mother reported Jennifer to be a slow eater, taking one hour for every bottle of 3 to 4 ounces. When this had not changed after one month, Mrs. E. became increasingly agitated and prepared herself for the feeds as if for a battle. She would use different nipples, add solids to the milk, hold the infant in various positions, and get extremely upset at the least bit of spitting up. These "vomits" she would measure and add to the next bottle. By 4 months Jennifer ate as poorly as ever and Mrs. E. spent virtually all day thinking about and preparing Jennifer's feeds. Despite all this effort, Jennifer weighed only 7 pounds 6 ounces at 5 months and feeding now took up to 12 hours a day. A month later Mrs. E. began placing a gastric tube down Jennifer's throat before most feeds. Yet Jennifer continued to vomit her feeds and gain weight poorly. Two months later Mrs. E.'s pediatrician finally asked for hospital admission. In hospital, Jennifer continued to eat little even when fed by the same competent nurse. She seemed to tense up as soon as she was picked up and put in a feeding position, turning her head away from the bottle as if to indicate her displeasure. As her weight remained stagnant, a gastrostomy was considered just prior to the psychiatric consultation.

During the consultation many conflictual issues between Mr. and Mrs. E. came to light. There was obvious marital discord, especially because of the anger both partners felt toward each other. Mrs. E. also appeared quite angry with Jennifer but found it difficult to acknowledge these feelings. There were also meetings with Jennifer's physicians and nurses, as well as observations of a number of feedings. These revealed Jennifer to be a very sensitive little girl who was easily disorganized when confronted with stimulation. She had also apparently learned to resent bottles and other containers of food although she related quite well to the examiner during her developmental assessment.

Since we felt that many of Jennifer's behaviors were reflections of her parents' feelings toward each other and toward her, the final treatment plan consisted of the following components: Mrs. E. was seen regularly by the psychiatrist to help her gain some control over her life. This meant more honest discussions with her husband, an increase in his involvement with Jennifer, and, after some months, the mother's part-time return to work. At the same time Jennifer was offered various bottles as toys, hoping that this would help in making bottles more acceptable to her. She was also given an opportunity to play with some other children who enjoyed being fed and whom she would watch during their meals quite eagerly. Jennifer herself was fed by two specifically designated nurses in a deliberately stereotypic and "distant" way as she seemed to be unable to cope with the massive stimulation her mother had brought upon her with each feeding. When this regime resulted in some improvement, Jennifer's mother, who had watched the initial feedings, began to feed the girl herself. When that proved possible, Jennifer was discharged home. There her mother initially continued to gavage feed her but was persuaded to give her one feed a day without the tube and increase this by one bottle feed a week. Mother was also told that the physical growth of her baby was the responsibility of her pediatrician and that insufficient weight gain did not reflect on her but on the pediatrician's competence. While progress was slow initially, Jennifer increasingly enjoyed her meals and three years later was a curious and intelligent preschooler although her weight remained at the fifth percentile.

SUMMARY

Feeding disorders are common in infants under 36 months of age and may be manifestations of difficulties in the early parent-child relationship. The majority of infants who have problems with eating will be treated by pediatricians but often in consultation with an infant mental health specialist. Specific subtypes of these disorders such as pica or ruminations can present a potentially life-threatening disorder and require urgent and thorough psychological assistance.

9

DISORDERS IN BEHAVIORAL ORGANIZATION

Historical Note

Researchers and clinicians have long observed differences in the reaction patterns of infants and young children to normal outside events. Some of these differences have been conceptualized as temperament (Thomas et al., 1963) and thereby regarded as legitimate variations of an infant's reactions to his or her surroundings. However, there are children who show such persistent extreme aberrations from the expected emotional or cognitive responses to everyday environmental events that they present a serious challenge to the average caretaker. In the past, the behavior of these children has been explained in various ways. For example, psychoanalysts have suggested that the strength of instinctual drives varies from one person to another and that this will affect the course of development. Hartmann (1958) in particular has discussed the importance of the inborn somatic and mental apparatus, which he called "autonomous ego functions," in the development of personality. He felt that these functions, which include muscle coordination, attention span, or musical ability, after appropriate differentiation, became important steering and control mechanisms for such attributes as perception, intentionality, the delay of affective discharges, and the synthesis of various other cognitive and emotional functions. Furthermore, Hartmann felt that a defect in any of these mechanisms could lead to a dyssynchrony between environmental demands and the organism's response to them.

Other psychoanalytically oriented clinicians who studied individual infants, referred because of developmentally inappropriate behaviors such as extreme shyness or heightened anxiety, suggested that such problems are related to unusual variations in drive development (Alpert et al., 1956). Escalona (1962; Bergmann & Escalona, 1949) presented convincing clinical examples of young infants who were so sensitive both physiologically and psychologically that ordinary stimuli seemed to overwhelm them.

While all these psychoanalytically oriented clinicians stress the biological, hence organic, vulnerability of these infants, others emphasized the importance of such innate differences in planning therapeutic measures for individual children (Provence & Lipton, 1962; Provence & Naylor, 1983).

More recently, a number of authors have discussed these apparently innate vulnerabilities in more ecological terms (Anders, 1978; Brazelton et al., 1974; Sander, 1975, 1980). These authors talk about the infant's innate ability to "organize" his or her behavior or state and discuss the impact specific caretaking routines may have in assisting an infant in the development or strategy for his or her biosocial adaptation. Despite the realization that these basic neurointegrative functions of the infant are important determinants of the child's day-to-day behavior, there are comparatively few writers who have discussed even the short-term behavioral consequences of infants born with apparent poor neuro-integration. Als and her group (Als, 1982; Als & Brazelton, 1981) have looked at premature infants and their negotiation of early organizational tasks. However, like Minde and his coworkers (1980), Als documented the difficulties such infants have in the smoothness and balance of their integrative functioning, the degree of modulation and regulation, and the effectiveness of their self-regulation only during the early months of life. Studies following such children into later childhood are clearly needed.

Clinical Description

The DSM-III classification does not include a condition that covers the cases subsumed under "Disorders in Behavioral Organization." The following diagnostic criteria are therefore presented as a preliminary description of this new category.

(A) Age of onset before 18 months.
(B) The child shows at least four of the following six categories:
    (1) The infant exhibits a general hyperreactivity to stimuli as shown by highly intense reactions to everyday events.

(2) The infant shows a lack of mechanisms that can modulate reactions to everyday events. This can take the form of:
   (a) Persistent crying or other expressions of unhappiness that the infant seems unable to control;
   (b) Excessive variations in emotional behavior and response to stimulation resulting from everyday caretaker-child interactions such as getting dressed, being put to bed, or being left alone in a room for brief periods.

(3) The infant shows a need for excessive cognitive or emotional stimulation for arousal that then may quickly lead to overexcitement and behavioral disorganization.

(4) The infant has had a history of unpredictable feeding pattern. This may be manifested by difficulties in establishing regular meal times or by an excessive variation of the infant's day-to-day food intake.

(5) The infant shows severe regressive anxiety and response to everyday stress. This may be manifested by a significant impairment of previously well-established cognitive or emotional milestones such as object constancy or self-other differentiation in response to a mild or moderate stress situation (e.g., a mild illness, the visits of guests to the house, etc.).

(6) The infant shows a grossly irregular sleeping pattern. He may have trouble falling asleep in the evening, may wake up frequently during the night, may have irregular nap times or engage in prolonged periods of head banging or other rhythmic activities while in bed.

(C) Not due to a physical disorder, mental retardation, or infantile autism.

(D) The difficulties have persisted for a minimum of 3 months.

The behavioral manifestations of the condition usually show themselves within the first 6 months of life. Infants at that time may have problems in organizing their sleep and wake patterns and only later show the behaviors described under Category B.

Infants with difficulties in behavioral organization usually show these problems through a variety of behavioral manifestations. For example, they may seem unable to soothe themselves before going to sleep by sucking their fingers or curling up into a ball in the corner of their crib. Instead, such infants may scream, flail their arms, and appear unable to move their extremities from an extension to a flexion position, which would provide them with much more control. At a later age such infants may also seemingly disintegrate (cry unconsolably or throw up their food) when faced with an unfamiliar event (such as a heavy rainfall or the first snow). They may take a long time to accommodate to the waking state after a nap (they may cry for some time whenever they wake up) and in general show highly sensitive and strong reponses to minimal external stimuli. A minor illness, for example, may set them back months in their cognitive or emotional development. Thus difficulties may relate to the apparently low threshold these babies show toward outside stimuli as well as the intensity with which they react to them.

During their second or third year of life, such children may have trouble retaining securely established cognitive achievements when they are challenged. For example, a 3-year-old boy may see a doll, bear, or tiger and be beside himself for fear that the small puppet may actually eat him or his mother. Such responses can often be elicited quite easily during a routine developmental or play assessment. Parents sometimes also report that these children seem to ask for punishment and even enjoy it. Thus they may ask for a spanking when they are in a disorganized state—as if the forceful parental intrusion into their behavior is the only possibility for them to get out of what they are doing.

Infants with this disorder are often presented to professionals as poor sleepers or poor eaters. On further inquiry the examiner may find that the total amount of sleep or food the infant has per day is quite adequate but that the distribution over 24 hours is unusual for his or her developmental stage. For example, a baby of 3 months may feed 30 or 40 times a day but rarely take more than one-half ounce per feed as he or she falls asleep whenever mother tries to give him more. Such an infant may also sleep in spurts of less than 30 minutes and may not have found a regular wake-sleep cycle even at 6 months. At 12 or 18 months such infants may also seemingly need to sleep with their mother or father as only by touching their bodies can they be reassured and put to sleep again after their night wakings. It is understandable that irregularities of this magnitude can lead to serious distortions in the general atmosphere at home and may cause severe strains in a marital relationship.

Infants who show sleeping or eating disorders without other signs of behavioral disorganization should be classified as presenting with developmental eating or sleeping disorders (see chapters 8 and 10).

Epidemiology

We have few data on the epidemiology of this disorder. Clinical reports about such children suggest that boys may be more often affected. The absolute frequency of this syndrome is unknown, although it is suggested that a certain percentage of children presently labeled as "feeding" or "sleeping" disorders in fact qualify for this syndrome. The histories of some children who are diagnosed as hyperactive at age 4 or 5 suggest similar early symptoms. Children of all socioeconomic groupings seem to be equally affected.

Etiology

We have no knowledge about any specific deficit that may be associated with this syndrome. However, there is some evidence that children who are born small for gestational age or prematurely are overrepresented in the clinical samples of such children (Als, 1983; Fitzhardinge & Stevens, 1974; Fitzhardinge, 1985). As the problems of these children could be conceptualized physiologically as a deficiency in the organizational or integrative aspect of the CNS one may well imagine that nutritional or other deficits in cerebral maturation may play a part in the etiology of the syndrome. On the other hand, clinical practice also suggests that infants who live in disorganized families and whose parents take little account of their emotional needs can display many of the symptoms of behavioral disorganization outlined in this chapter.

Differential Diagnosis

All conditions that can lead to sleep or eating disorders (see also chapters 8 and 10) must be ruled out. Usually, however, these disorders affect only one area of the infant's functioning. Some behavioral disorganization frequently occurs even in otherwise normal infants after major stresses such as hospitalization or the loss of a parent. However, both the degree and the duration of these disturbances will be much less pervasive and respond well to short-term supportive external measures.

Disturbances in autonomic regulation can also be caused by certain medical conditions. For example, mental retardation or the sequelae of encephalitis and other traumatic or toxic events leading to brain injury may simulate many of the symptoms described under this syndrome. They can be ruled out with the help of neurological examination or an EEG or specific psychological tests.

Children with a "difficult" temperament can exhibit some of the characteristics of such a child. However, in contrast to these children a youngster with problems in behavioral organization will show his or her difficulties primarily when stressed but not as a habitual way of interacting with the world.

Some autistic children may exhibit symptoms suggestive of behavioral disorganization. A more detailed history will reveal, however, that the biological and language functions of these children are affected along with their emotional, cognitive, or social development.

Prognosis

The duration and outcome of the condition has not been established but appears to be variable. In the majority of cases the child will finally "find his or her way in the world" and adjust to the realities of his or her existence, especially if the infant's caregivers can provide the structure and support the infant has difficulties in generating himself or herself. This will usually not happen before the second or third year of life and may not be totally successful until middle childhood for a substantial minority of children. It is obvious that infants with serious manifestations of the disorder will present a severe challenge to the best intentioned, competent, ordinary caretaker. Some of these children may develop learning disorders with their associated social problems later in life, or have a higher incidence of hyperactivity or psychosomatic illnesses and remain more vulnerable to external stresses.

Treatment

Treatment of a child who has problems in behavioral organization should include a thorough medical and psychological examination to rule out any possible biological disorder or mental retardation. While traditionally investigators have feared that parents may be hurt when they are told about a neurological disorder, recent work suggests that most parents "know" about their child's deficit up to 6 months before the average physician can objectively diagnose it (Minde & Perrotta, 1985). This suggests that even in the absence of specific remedies, the knowledge parents may gain from discussing their fears about their child's disability with a professional can be helpful and reassuring to them.

The psychological treatment of this condition must aim at helping both the parents and the baby. Parents should first be reassured about their baby's basic cognitive competence and told about the syndrome in detail. The goal here is to make them into experts at "reading" their infant and responding appropriately. While detailed programs depend on the defects of a particular infant, the clinician may demonstrate strategies to soothe and/or organize such an infant. For example, a baby who cannot calm himself or herself at night may need to be swaddled or put in his or her crib in a curled up position with a blanket over the crib to cut out unnecessary stimuli. As carrying around such distressed and crying babies will expose them to more stimulation, which they cannot handle, it is usually best to put such an infant down or hold them quietly in a dark room. In general, these children do best with strict routines, well-developed bed- and bathtime rituals, and ample time to adjust to any changes in their day-to-day life (such as a new babysitter). Pacifiers may be of great help to such infants as a focus of behavioral organization.

It is obvious that therapeutic suggestions have to be tailored to each infant-caretaker dyad. However, we usually begin our work by trying to help these children with the organization of their biological irregularities (such as sleeping and eating) so as to provide a predictable basis on which their overall behavior can be anchored. Good mothers have often developed ingenious ways of calming and regulating their infants that should be reinforced and built on. Much will also depend on the clinician's impression about the present interactional adequacy of baby and caretaker. With experience the clinician can get to understand the needs of such difficult infants quite quickly and provide some behavioral assistance right before a watching mother. For example, a little 2-year-old boy may be too frightened to touch a new toy but may be able to point to it in the mirror. Such an interchange can teach a mother that her infant needs "buffers" in his dealing with the world and can help her think of other ways to increase his spectrum of behavioral modulations. If a mother is too insensitive or preoccupied with her own concerns, the clinician may either look for more sensitive caretaker substitutes, such as the father, a relative, or sibling, to teach them about the condition or try to learn more about why the mother is limited in her responsiveness to her infant. Some easily disorganized children may also benefit from special nursery settings in which well-trained personnel can help them to build up more solid behavioral structures.

In summary, the treatment of children with disturbances in behavioral organization is as complex as are the syndrome's behavioral manifestations. Expert knowledge of normal child development and sensitive caretaker-child observations are the key to successful intervention.

CASE EXAMPLE

Case 4

Gillian G. was 18 months old when she was first referred for psychiatric assessment. Her father, a 34-year-old lawyer, and her mother, a 29-year-old former nursery school teacher, were both puzzled and frustrated by a number of behaviors Gillian displayed. For example, Gillian had never slept through the night but during the first 14 months of her life seemed to have been content to lie in her bed quietly. This was witnessed by her mother, who had checked her at all hours of the night and always found her silently awake in the same position in which she had been placed in her crib. However, some 3 months before seeing the clinician, Gillian had suddenly begun to cry at night "as if she had discovered that one could do something about this nightly loneliness." Since then the parents had tried various ways of consoling Gillian but found that the only successful way was for the mother to move into her room and sleep on a mattress that Gillian could see from her crib. Her mother, in fact, reported that while her sleeping on the floor kept Gillian calm during the night, on awakening she would invariably find Gillian looking at her in a "solemn, worried fashion." Other unusual behaviors had to do with a white rug that her parents had designated "hers" when she was 6 months old and on which most of her toys were placed. While Gillian was perfectly mobile she would often stand on the edge of this rug crying bitterly "as if she thought she was surrounded by deep water."

Gillian's past history revealed her to be the first-born child of her parents. Her mother had an uneventful, wanted pregnancy but had gone into premature labor six weeks before term. Gillian's birthweight was only 1280 grams, about 400 grams less than would have been expected in a 34-week gestation baby. Yet in hospital Gillian gained weight rapidly, ate well, and was home after six weeks. There, both parents were keen to make up for the time she had lost in hospital and provided the little girl with abundant love and stimulation. Gillian seemed to enjoy this care, was cuddly and responsive but from early on tried to keep one of her parents in sight at all times. As the G. family seemed to have such a good time together, her mother hardly noticed that Gillian from the day of her discharge from hospital did not have a daytime nap and even in the evening would not seem to settle down until 11 p.m. or later.

Gillian's general development was quite precocious. She sat at 5 months, walked by herself at 10 months, and had sentences of 3 to 4 words by the time of her initial consultation. Assessment in fine motor and adaptive skills had her pass all 24-month and some 30-month items (such as drawing a cross, building a tower of nine cubes). Yet she did not seem to relish her accomplishments but appeared almost driven to finish each task. When the doctor tried to play with her, she did not leave her mother's lap nor look at the examiner during the first 30 minutes. Later on, the examiner noticed that she did not touch the small animal figures she had not seen before (a zebra and lion) although she could identify them in the pictures in a book she had brought along. However, in the second session at her house she seemed generally more relaxed and at ease and happy to relate to the examiner from her white rug.

Ten months later there were new developments. Her father, who had begun to take Gillian to the local zoo on Sunday mornings so as to provide her with a pleasant routine, had found this to become an increasingly frustrating experience. The girl would anxiously anticipate the zoo visit, could hardly be contained until she had seen "her" bear, lion, or elephant, and would become increasingly agitated when her father could not get to the respective pavilions quickly. There had also been a two-hour crying spell when a waitress in a McDonald's who normally served Mr. G. and Gillian during their Sunday outings had been away on vacation. Her mother also reported new problems with activities such as birthday parties when Gillian appeared very eager to go but once on the way would get scared and scream to go home again.

SUMMARY

Disorders of behavioral organization are relatively common manifestations during early infancy. They affect aspects of the emotional and cognitive development of an infant, showing themselves in disturbances of sleeping, eating, autonomic control, modulation of affect, or other integrative behavioral functions. They seem to occur more commonly in children who have experienced premature birth, were born small for gestational age, or had other illnesses affecting the CNS. Treatment must be directed at assisting these infants in their attempts to regulate their behavior and may involve intensive work with caretakers.

10

SLEEP DISORDERS

A sleep disorder in infancy is characterized by either an excess or deficit of sleeping time, disturbances in the sleep pattern, also called "parasomnia," or a difficulty in settling down to sleep.

Historical Note

Difficulties in sleeping have long been described in young children. However, following the observation by Aserinsky and Kleitman (1953) that sleep can occur during at least two distinct states of CNS organization, the REM and the non-REM state, investigators have become far more knowledgeable about the developmental changes of sleep patterns in infants. For example, Parmelee (1964) provided ontogenetic data on the normal sleep pattern of infants from birth to 16 weeks. He described a number of distinct shifts in sleep organization during infancy that were further developed by Anders and his group. The highlights of these data are as follows:

(1) The time a sleeping infant spends in the REM state decreases from 60% of sleep time at birth to 43% at 3 months and 30% of total sleep time by 1 year (Anders, 1982).
(2) The infant enters sleep via the REM state at birth. This pattern is replaced during the latter part of the first year by the adult pattern of entering a non-REM state first.
(3) REM states alternate with non-REM states in the newborn all through his or her sleep time. At about 6 months, they move to the later parts of the sleep period, again approximating the adult pattern.
(4) Concomitant to these physiological changes, infants gain increasing control over their state organization by 3 months. Thus 70% of normal infants sleep through the night by 3 months and 90% by 9 months (Moore & Ucko, 1957).

While sleep difficulties in infancy have long been described their reliable measurement and the measurement of their incidence have only recently been possible. The reasons are twofold. Parental reports of sleep problems may be inaccurate as parents often report only the time when an infant wakes up but leave out when he or she went to bed. That is, an infant who sleeps from 7 p.m. to 2 a.m. is labeled as a "night waker," while the baby who sleeps from 10:30 p.m. to 5:30 a.m. is considered to "sleep through" although both infants sleep seven hours. Furthermore, there are many parents who do not feel disturbed by their children's night waking. Yet traditional EEG recordings are so cumbersome and stress inducing that they may distort subsequent sleep patterns. However, the recently developed time-lapse video recording of sleep-wake behavior in infants (Anders & Sostek, 1976) has allowed very precise measurements of an infant's behavior at night. Among other things, it has documented that about 80% of all infants aged 12 months wake up at night for short periods but that about 60% of those who do wake up lie quietly in bed and go back to sleep without making any fuss. There are also no reliable data available that correlate infants' behavior at night with their daytime activities or the type of relationship they have with their caretakers.

Clinical Description

Disorders in the organization or duration of sleep are not at present part of the DSM-III diagnostic manual although sleep disturbances such as sleepwalking (307.46) or night terrors (307.49) are discussed in the manual. However, the Sleep Disorders Classification Committee of the Association of Sleep Disorder Centres and the Association of the Psychophysiological Study of Sleep (Roffwarg et al., 1979) published an outline of a diagnostic classification system of sleep and arousal disorders. While this classification includes disorders that do not occur in infants, it does describe the following syndromes applicable to this age group.

(A) Disorders of Initiating and Maintaining Sleep
    (1) Transient and situational
    (2) Persistent

A precise definition of this term is not given in the manual. However, Richman and her group (Richman, 1981) defined a sleep disorder as a problem that existed for more than 3 months with 5 or more nights a week of awakening. In addition, a severe sleep disorder was characterized by one or more of the following:

(1) waking 3 or more times a night, or
(2) waking for more than 20 minutes during the night, or
(3) being taken into the parents' bed.

A settling disorder was defined as any child who fails to fall asleep within 30 minutes after being put to bed.

(B) Disorders of Excessive Somnolence
(1) Transient
(2) Persistent

A child would be given this diagnosis if his or her sleep had increased by more than 25% from his or her own baseline for more than one month.

(C) Disorders of Sleep-Wake Cycle
(1) Transient
(2) Persistent

This disorder can be expressed by either a frequently changing sleep-wake cycle or by an irregular sleep-wake pattern of the infant for more than one month.

Infants may find it difficult to fall asleep at appropriate times or they may wake at several times during the night. As mentioned above, infants normally develop a regular sleep-wake rhythm by 3 to 4 months of age and will sleep for a consecutive period of nine hours during the night. An infant who has not developed such a pattern by 6 months and wakes up more than three nights a week for more than one month should be given such a diagnosis. Transient disorders should cover children affected for one to two months, persistent disorders for those who have shown the behavior for a longer period.

Some infants show an apparently excessive need for sleep both at night and during the day (that is, will increase their sleeping time by 25% or more in a comparatively short period). Clinically, such children are usually poorly cared for at home or placed in overcrowded daycare centers where the staff has little time or inclination to provide adequate stimulation. As such, caretakers often inadvertently welcome the sleepy baby because "he doesn't make much trouble." The condition is often not recognized and the infant is not referred for the appropriate professional help.

Some infants present with persistently irregular sleep-wake patterns or frequently changing sleep-wake cycles. Such infants may sleep sufficiently long stretches of time but do so at varying times during the day or night. They may also sleep for excessive periods and then be awake for 12 or 15 hours.

Epidemiology

Sleep disorders, especially those presenting as problems of initiating and maintaining sleep, are among the most common disorders in young children. Epidemiological studies of neurologically normal full-term infants show that 30% of children do not sleep through the hours of midnight and 5 a.m. by 3 months of age, 17% by 6 months, and 10% by 12 months (Moore and Ucko, 1957). Carey (1970), who reported on more than 200 infants in his private practice, found that 18% of his patients awoke regularly at 6 months. Bernal (1972), who examined a group of 77 medically low-risk infants at 14 months, identified 24 infants (31%) as showing disturbances of frequent night waking. When the same group was reexamined around their third birthday, 40% were still described as waking more than one night a week and about 80% of those were in the problem group at 14 months. This suggests that a good number of infants with sleeping problems do not outgrow this difficulty within the first 3 years.

In the most comprehensive study of sleep disorders, Richman and associates (1982) examined 705 3-year-old youngsters in a London borough and followed a representative subsample of 283 children to age 8. At 3 years 16.0% of these youngsters had difficulty settling and 14.5% woke up at least three times a week. At 4 years 15% still woke up 3 or more times a week and 12% still could not settle. When Richman and her colleagues (Richman et al., 1982) compared a subgroup of 94 behavior-disordered with 91 matched control children at age 3, the rate of difficulties for settling as well as waking disorders was higher (28.7%) among the behavior-disordered children. At age 8, two-thirds of the control and all of the behavior-disordered children who had displayed difficulties in settling at age 3 still showed these problems. In fact, difficulty in settling at night showed the second highest consistency out of 20 behaviors between the ages of 3 and 8 (Richman et al., 1982, p. 91). This suggests that later problem sleepers can be identified early on in life although a majority of poor sleepers will outgrow their difficulties before the age of 3.

Etiology

The etiology of sleeping disorders is not easily known. While the Association of Sleep Disorders Centres defines the disorders of initiating and maintaining sleep as psychophysiological—that is, biological in nature—there are no data that prove this association. In fact, there is good evidence that both biological vulnerabilities and psychological difficulties within the family are associated with poor sleeping. For example, Richman (1981), in a study that examined 77 nonreferred infants age 1 to 2 years in a London borough, found 9.5% to suffer from a "severe waking problem." When she compared this group with a normal control sample, 55% of the waking versus 27% of the control children (p < .05) also had behavior problems and 40% versus 17% (p < .05) had been in accidents requiring medical care. Furthermore, in 51% versus 17% (p < .01) the mothers showed a psychiatric problem and 31% versus none had a significantly elevated malaise score. On the other hand, 30% of the waking versus 16% (p < .05) of the control children also had a history of severe adverse perinatal events.

In a more recent study Richman (1985) reported 33% of the mothers of severely sleep-disordered children to show mild neurotic symptoms and not to confide in their husbands. Lozoff and his colleagues (Lozoff et al., 1985), in a very recent epidemiological investigation, also found that mothers of sleep-disordered youngsters were rated as more ambivalent (85% versus 35%) and had experienced more life events (8.8% versus 6.3%). They were also more often diagnosed to show a depressed mood (46% versus 19%).

While parental anxiety and depression may well influence an infant's sleeping pattern because anxious parents may sleep less and be more likely to hear their child at night, there have been no prospective studies that demonstrate how a parent's behavior actually influences an infant's sleep pattern. On the other hand, there is some evidence that specific temperamental dispositions and neonatal events might predispose some children to wake up more easily than others and thereby make them more likely to show sleep disorders. For example, Carey (1970) suggested that in his sample a significantly higher number of infants who had sleeping problems at 6 months had a difficult temperament than did their nonaffected peers. In addition, Blurton-Jones (1978) found a high association between night waking and suboptimal obstetric events. Richman and her group (Richman, 1981; Richman et al., 1985) also reported that about one-third of their poor sleepers had a history of cesarean section, transient asphyxia, or other perinatal complications.

Excessive somnolence, as was pointed out earlier, is generally related to lack of stimulation and poor psychosocial milieu of an infant. It is as if the infant wanted to escape the boredom and neglect by regressing into sleep. However, here again some biological predisposition may determine why one understimulated infant will sleep much while another becomes aggressive or depressed.

Differential Diagnosis

Sleeping disorders must be differentiated from attachment disorders and disorders of behavioral organization. Children who are anxiously attached may also be afraid to go to sleep at night as they fear that their mothers may leave them. Such children often refuse to be put down in their cribs and will only fall asleep while being carried about. However, they will also show other classical symptoms of separation anxiety or conflict.

Children with disorders of behavioral organization may also show irregular sleeping patterns. However, these children usually also exhibit difficulties in their affective behavior and may present other prolems of CNS organization.

Many young children will exhibit transient sleep disturbances in response to anxiety-provoking experiences such as moving into a new bed, a visit to grandmother, or the birth of a new baby. These disturbances often last a few days only and should not be given a psychiatric diagnosis. Sleep disorders in rare cases can also be a reflection of epileptic disturbance or a sign of a severe CNS disorder. A neurological and/or EEG examination will usually be sufficient to clarify the diagnosis.

Prognosis

Sleep disorders may range from mild to severe and persist for varying lengths of time. While few authors have followed children with sleeping problems for long periods, there is some evidence from one study (Richman et al., 1982) that at least 17% of the children who have this disorder at 3 years still do not sleep through the night by age 8. A cluster analysis of the same cohort of 183 children in the study by Richman and her associates showed that at age 8 the children with the sleep disorders also tended to be difficult to control and had a poor appetite and faddy eating habits. Wolkind and Everitt (1974) in a study examining 3-year-olds who attended nursery schools and were in "special care" also identified a cluster of children with both sleeping and eating disorders as well as specific fears and habits. This suggests that sleep disorders in later childhood are frequently associated with other symptoms of psychopathology and may at times be precursors of a later neurotic or emotional disturbance. When poor sleep organization is part of a child's generally poor behavioral organization, one may see later disturbances in the organization or control of affect.

Treatment

The treatment of sleeping disorders must be tailored to the perceived origin of the difficulties. For example, parents whose focus on an infant's sleep pattern is extreme, who are anxious and perceive any crying after the infant has been put down as a sign of their poor parenting abilities, must be encouraged to give their infant time to settle down. In cases where a baby seems to be hyperactive, ways must be found to calm the infant before he or she settles for bed. As a general strategy for the treatment of sleep disorders, however, it is useful to ask parents to keep a detailed log of their child's sleeping behavior for one week. They should record the time the infant went to bed, how long it took the infant to fall asleep, the average total time the child slept at night, and the number of wakings per night. Parents should also report the hours he or she spent in their bed per week. Richman and her group (1981) have found that a discussion of this log will often demonstrate that the child in fact gets enough sleep over a 24-hour period, which in itself may reassure the parents. Such a log also helps in pointing out effective parental management strategies and provides a good baseline for the evaluation of interventions that have been suggested by the clinician.

While a detailed review of behavioral management techniques of sleep disorders is beyond the scope of this volume, a general approach should contain the following elements.

(1) Young children like to feel in charge over some aspect of their environment. This can best be achieved by providing them with regular routines that allow them to predict the next event from the preceding activity and thus permit them to feel "in control." Bedtime should therefore be at approximately the same time each day and should be preceded by some rituals. These may consist of a song, a short story, or kisses for the dolls given each day in the same order.

(2) Children who do not want to or cannot sleep immediately should be given the option of playing in bed. They should not, however, be allowed to get out of bed again and disturb their parents.

(3) When children seem very anxious at being left alone in their bedroom, a parent may remain in the room but not interact with the child. This will assure the child but at the same time avoid parental manipulation. The parent may then gradually move out of the room—sit farther and farther away from the child in the course of a week or 10 days and in that way help the child to sleep by him- or herself.

(4) Children who have learned to control their families through crying at bedtime may have to be left to "cry it out" for up to 30 or even 45 minutes. While this may seem to be a rather heartless form of treatment, it will work within two or three days in more than 80% of all cases.

However, it should be stressed that a certain number of sleep disorders are a reflection of parental conflicts and may not respond to such behavioral suggestions. Thus there are mothers who "must check" on their baby or youngster every 15 minutes after he or she is put in bed. This may be disturbing for the infant and create sleeping problems. Marital conflicts also often spill over into bedtime routines. For example, there may be a competition about which parent says goodnight last and hence is most loved by the child. These things must be addressed in meetings with the parents and counseling may be necessary. Some children also have such poor state regulation that they need to be helped to settle very slowly by gradually dimming the light or playing specific music. It is obvious that such treatment plans must be thought out carefully and must take account of both the psychological and behavioral aspects and needs of the child and his or her family. Sedatives should not be given to induce sleep in young children as virtually all of them disrupt normal REM sleep and subsequent waking behavior (Richman, 1985).

Problems of hypersomnia are treated by providing the infant with adequate stimulation and care. Placing a child into bed should also never be used as a method of punishment or constraint since this double role of the bed as a place for punishment as well as peaceful sleep confuses the child and creates more difficulties in sleeping.

CASE EXAMPLE

Case 5

Mrs. P., a 26-year-old secretary, and her 14-month-old boy Jeremy were referred to the child psychiatric clinic by her general practitioner because she felt that the infant cried so much at night that his mother seemed incapable of handling him any more. In addition, Jeremy would spend up to two hours each evening and night banging his head against his crib, which upset both his parents. On examination, Mrs. P. gave a long history of difficulties with Jeremy, her only child. The boy was born following an emergency cesarean section because of poor fetal heart sounds. This had made mother feel "very guilty for not making his entry into life more easy." After 10 days in hospital Jeremy had come home with his mother but "right away turned day into night." Thus he would sleep in the morning and afternoon but be up by 7 p.m. and allegedly stay up most of the night. While mother carried him around a lot during these early months nevertheless he would cry a good deal, waking up his father and causing arguments between the parents. Things got worse two months prior to the consultation, when Jeremy, after having cried for about 30 minutes, commenced to bang his head against the end of his bed. This would last up to 45 minutes and be repeated whenever he woke up during the night.

His mother had tried to pad the sides of his bed, but Jeremy had pried the padding away and almost seemed to enjoy the bangings of his head. Mother was so upset about this that she tried to calm Jeremy by setting up tapes of music and her voice in his bedroom. However, this had not stopped the crying or head banging and still necessitated mother to carry Jeremy around during much of the night.

Mr. P., who did not help his wife in the night ministrations, always felt that Jeremy should be left alone at night and not be attended to when he cried. Since Jeremy had screamed for more than 45 minutes on several occasions when Mrs. P. had tried to let him "cry it out," this approach seemed irresponsible and potentially harmful to mother. The difference of opinion about the management of Jeremy's sleeping problem between Mr. and Mrs. P. had become so focused that Mr. P., two weeks prior to the appointment, had threatened to leave Mrs. P. if she "couldn't get Jeremy's sleeping behavior under control within the next month," giving the final impetus for the consultation.

Further interviews with Mrs. P. alone and with both parents revealed that the mother came from a family where women were generally devalued, while the father, the owner of a pharmacy, as an only son had always been adored by his mother. The father also stated that he had been hyperactive as a youngster and was given Ritalin for 10 years and still found it hard not to have his way.

Jeremy showed many signs of a difficult temperament. Thus he had a low threshold to any type of stimulation, was quite active, concentrated little on any task, and was easily upset. A detailed sleep analysis also revealed that he was usually up for only 30 to 40 minutes at night whenever he cried. As he still had two daytime naps, he in fact obtained sufficient sleep. Since Jeremy's sleeping problem appeared to be the result of temperamental as well as intrafamilial difficulties, treatment focused on both these areas. In particular, the mother was instructed to bathe Jeremy before his bedtime, then dry him in his room with only one light on, sing him two songs, and then leave him alone. If he cried or banged his head he was to be left for 10 minutes at first, after which his mother would come in to stand next to him and touch his body but not talk to him. If he cried again his mother would come only after 15 minutes and repeat the procedure. By the next time she came only after Jeremy had cried for 20 minutes, and so on. In addition, his mother was seen alone by a psychiatrist to provide her with more confidence in herself. Once this had been achieved, her husband was included in the discussions.

Follow-up revealed that Jeremy stopped his crying within three weeks but continued to bang his head for brief periods before falling asleep. Mother became more assertive toward both Jeremy and her husband and the latter, after many discussions, adapted to his "new" wife.

SUMMARY

Sleeping disorders are among the most common problems in early childhood. While initially infants with sleeping problems wake up a number of times at night, during the second and third year the symptomatology often shifts to difficulties these children have in settling down at night. There is also evidence that 20% of children with sleeping problems at age 3 still show sleeping or emotional problems at age 8. Finally, there are also good data that suggest that a significant number of sleeping problems are the result of both biological vulnerabilities of the child and problems within their families. Treatment must therefore include work with both the family and the child.

11

TREATMENT

In the preceding chapters we have outlined some treatment approaches appropriate for specific disturbances in infants. When we now devote an entire chapter to psychiatric intervention methods in infancy, we pursue two goals. One is to take stock of the concepts and principles mental health specialists have developed about the treatment of infants. This will also allow us to clarify some of the potential misunderstandings surrounding such terms as "infant stimulation" or "psychotherapy in infancy." The other goal is to discuss the different methods used to treat infants and their respective efficacy. This will also permit us to deal with the frequently expressed opinion that infants will grow out of their problems because of their developmental plasticity and that treatment in such young, immature organisms is both impracticable and invalid.

The reader should be aware that this chapter will not deal with pharmacological or other biological measures that can help infants in their general functioning. Such treatment forms have been discussed in the chapters that dealt with specific psychiatric conditions. The present chapter therefore will focus primarily on the treatment of those disorders that occur in infants with presumably normal innate capacities.

PRINCIPLES GOVERNING THE TREATMENT OF INFANTS

The specific principles governing the treatment of infants and their families have varied widely among individual clinicians. However, in the most general terms therapists have always aimed at assisting their small patients in their general development, helping the infant to be active motorically, socially, affectively, and intellectually (Provence, 1983). In fact, it has been stated that therapy that enables an infant to interact with the outside world will often lead to a reduction or disappearance of symptomatic problems (Provence, 1974).

Mahrer and associates (1976), in a theoretical discussion of infant psychotherapy, saw the goals of such treatment to be an enhanced selfhood, more behavioral control, and more self-competence of the infant. These outcome criteria have been elaborated on in more detail by White (1959), Moss (1967), and Mahler and her group (1975), as well as by Yarrow and his colleagues (1976). Furthermore, all these authors underscore the fundamental premise of therapy with infants—namely, that treatment goals cannot be presumed to occur automatically through an unfolding of stages of maturation but need the presence of nurturing adults for their actualization (Provence, 1972).

There are five basic principles that have been guiding therapists:

(1) The infant's relationship to a nurturing adult is of fundamental importance to his or her unencumbered development. It is therefore essential that parents or other caretakers be helped to carry out the necessary nurturing functions at least reasonably well.

Both general developmental and psychoanalytic theories have long stressed that close ties of trust and love between an infant and his or her parents play a central role in his or her emotional and cognitive development. Therefore we feel that any treatment that fails to acknowledge the importance of this relationship cannot be called therapeutic.

(2) Infants, because of their general immaturity, present far more global disturbances in response to specific bodily illnesses or noxious psychosocial experiences than do older children.

This is in concert with the principle that the development moves from a relatively global to a more differentiated functional state (Werner, 1940). Therefore, therapy cannot consist of stimulating only the most obviously disturbed developmental function but must always consider the infant's total interpersonal, social, and physical needs.

(3) Good psychological care of an infant includes care of his or her physical as well as cognitive and emotional needs.

Most infant mental health workers agree on the importance the affective atmosphere and varied stimuli and challenges have for the infant's development. However, the care of an infant's body, as Provence (1972) has pointed out, is of equal therapeutic importance for two reasons. On the one hand, the provision of an adequate diet, proper clothing, and immunizations, as well as the symptomatic treatment of physical disorders, are part of the interventions expected of every health professional. On the other hand, we also know that the care given to the body early on in life also affects the infant's beginning awareness of his or her body and through it his or her sense of mastery vis-à-vis the outside world. Being bathed or touched tenderly cleans the body but also communicates interest or protectiveness and in this way contributes significantly to the experience of pleasure and well-being.

(4) Problems in development are usually the result of both innate and experiential factors.

While this might appear obvious to most readers, it is not always considered when treatment plans are developed. A careful history and evaluation as outlined in Chapter 3, delineating both the strength and vulnerabilities of the infant and his or her caretaking environment, is therefore necessary before any intervention is planned.

(5) Babies need both freedom for their self-initiated activities and age-appropriate limits or prohibitions.

Opportunities to play and take the lead in interactions are obvious ingredients of an infant's development agenda, especially after the age of 6 months. However, infants are also born with the capacity to learn to postpone gratification and to tolerate tension. Infants who have been deprived or neglected may not reveal their poor capacity for self-regulation until these primary deficits are at least partially corrected. A therapeutic approach that concentrates solely on giving and providing, however, may fail to see the need an infant may also have for judicious limits and frustrations.

METHODS OF TREATMENT

The foregoing principles of infant therapy have been put into practice by clinicians using a variety of therapeutic modalities. In the present section we will examine those modalities that have been most popular. Dividing them into direct and indirect treatment methods, we will discuss studies or clinical reports that have examined their efficacy to assess the advantages and disadvantages of specific approaches to the treatment of infants and their caretakers.

DIRECT TREATMENT

Psychoanalysis

Sigmund Freud's treatment of little Hans through his father (S. Freud, 1909) was the first recorded psychological treatment of a preschooler. Freud's hope that the early direct treatment of children would assist their later development was shared by many of his early followers. Thus, there are a number of reports of infant analyses by early psychoanalysts (see Bornstein, 1935; Sterba, 1949; Schwartz, 1950; Fraiberg, 1952; Sperling, 1952; Leonard, 1959; Klein, 1960). However, the majority of psychoanalysts have refrained from analyzing infants. For example, A. Freud (1945, 1968) in her articles dealing with the indications for child analysis, does not recommend this form of treatment for such young children because they do not yet show "internalized conflicts." Neubauer (1972) agrees with A. Freud, stating that in order to analyze children, a therapeutic alliance has to be formed that must have two components—forming a relationship and making it work for the therapeutic aim. This, according to Neubauer, can only be achieved if the child has gone through the separation-individuation phase of development and has a distinct sense of him- or herself and others (object constancy). As these developmental criteria are not usually met before the age of 2½, one can generally say that psychoanalytic treatment for infants is not indicated. However, as will be pointed out later in this chapter, psychoanalytic theory has been one of the most important underpinnings of much therapeutic guidance provided for families of infants and toddlers.

BEHAVIORAL TREATMENT

The behavioral remediation of specific symptoms in infants has been used for some 60 years. Stimulated by Watson and Rayner's classical paper on the conditioned emotional response (1920), Jones (1924) reported on the treatment of severe fear reactions in young children, claiming that conditioning and social imitation were effective although other behavioral methods were not.

Later attempts to use behavior modification techniques in the treatment of infants were aimed at specific behaviors such as temper tantrums at bedtime (Williams, 1959) or water phobias (Bentler, 1962). Although these authors were very specific about their methodology, a contemporary reader of their papers will be struck by the total disregard these authors had for the possible dynamics underlying their young patients' problems. For example, the 21-month-old infant in Williams's study (Williams, 1959) had been ill for about 18 months and experienced frequent hospitalizations. After his final recovery he continued to be fearful and began to cry at the suggestion of being put to bed. The possibility that this infant may have displayed a developmentally highly appropriate fear of a possible renewed abandonment by his mother at bedtime was never discussed in Williams's paper. This suggests that early behaviorists, much like the early psychoanalysts, were rather narrow in the application of their theoretical model to the treatment of young children. More recent work (Berkowitz & Graziano, 1972; Schaefer & Millman, 1977), however, provides evidence that present-day behavioral therapists use a far more developmentally and dynamically sensitive approach when treating young children.

The Mother as Therapist of the Infant

Realizing that parents are an infant's most constant human partners, clinicians have long attempted to train mothers to be their children's therapists. The best-known form of "filial therapy" has been developed by Guerney and his group (Guerney, 1964; Andronico et al., 1967). Guerney described a four- to eight-week course where play techniques are demonstrated to a group of mothers who then begin to "practice" on their own or the teaching staff's children. Group sessions continue after the two months of training in the form of supervisory seminars to which mothers bring the material they have encountered with their own patient children to the group for discussion. It is of interest that some 10 years earlier Carl Rogers suggested an almost identical approach to his daughter, whose 18-month-old infant was terrified of having a bowel movement and/or her diapers changed (Fuchs, 1957). In an exchange of letters published by Mrs. Fuchs, Rogers suggested that she buy some specific toys, put them in a designated box, and play with her daughter every day for 45 minutes in a special place in the home. Mrs. Fuchs describes this method as having eliminated her daughter's symptoms within two weeks.

Johnson and associates (1980), in a more recent essay, reported on more than 100 mothers whose infants presented irregularities of sleeping or feeding and general adjustment problems, shown by clinging, temper tantrums, or unhappiness. According to Johnson, mothers met in groups of 10, together with their infants, once a month for a short discussion and instructional session. The mothers then spent 30 minutes in a small room under supervision where they consciously encouraged their infants to take an interactional lead and followed their behavior as unobtrusively as possible. The mothers continued these types of sessions every day at home and later used the monthly meetings to obtain feedback and suggestions from other mothers and the group leaders.

These forms of treatment seem to be designed to sensitize mothers to their infants' state, competence, and feelings. Although no formal studies have evaluated the effect of such endeavors, it seems likely that at least some mothers can be trained to be effective therapists of their infants provided they have few personal conflicts and no need to be in charge. On the basis of our therapeutic principles, we would suggest that any encouragement of "activity" in an infant is usually beneficial, although infants need the experience of both leading and being led. While the emphasis in filial therapy on a basically passive but one hopes contingent caretaker may benefit children whose need for autonomy and competence has not been sufficiently recognized, other infants may require a more diverse intervention to overcome their behavioral difficulties.

INDIRECT TREATMENT

Clinicians using an indirect treatment modality serve as counselors for the primary caretaker or other adults who are in frequent contact with a disturbed or troubled infant. The rationale for this approach is the notion, best expressed by Jacobs (1949), that mothers regard infants as part of themselves and are consequently readily engaged in counseling. As the developing relationship between the primary caretaker and the infant forms the basis of all later relationships of this infant, the importance of the direct treatment approach can hardly be overstated. However, as a number of distinct indirect counseling techniques have been developed, a more precise description of the concepts underlying these procedures seems in order.

Dynamic or Reflective Counseling

Therapists subscribing to this type of counseling are frequently influenced by psychoanalytic and other dynamic child development theories. They believe that mothers and other key people in the infant's world should be helped to understand the developmental needs of their infants so that they may provide them with the required stimulation and care.

While the actual process of sensitizing caretakers to the needs of their children varies from practitioner to practitioner, the majority of counseling therapists avoid suggesting any direct action to their clients. Instead, they see their role in assisting the adults to improve their abilities to reflect and conceptualize their infant's behavior. Furthermore, such therapists aim to help parents clarify their own goals as well as the needs expressed in the symptoms of their children (Auerbach, 1968). Detailed accounts of such counseling programs have been given by Friedlander (1946) and Jacobs (1949). Both these authors also emphasize that they would not deal with the personal problems of the children's mothers nor see the troubled infants themselves.

In contrast, a number of authors have claimed that it is the combination of parental counseling and direct work with young children that is the most effective treatment. For example, A. Freud (1954) urged that mothers be taught how to use their selective influence on the infant's constitutional endowment to stimulate and encourage those things that would further development and discourage regression. While Freud implied that this work with parents should go on individually, others have taken the concept further. Thus Alpert (1959, 1967) assembled up to five infants and their mothers twice weekly for one hour in a nursery setting. Mothers had a chance to observe their infants at play and discuss issues of concern with the teachers and a psychiatrist. Unfortunately, neither Friedlander, Jacobs, nor Alpert provide any data on the duration and outcome of their respective treatment procedures.

S. Fraiberg, whose initial training as a social worker undoubtedly influenced her approach, is probably the most outspoken advocate of involving the whole family in an infant's treatment. In an early paper (1950) she exemplified her method of intervention using a group of infants with sleep disturbance. She stated that infants whose problems were detected very early could be treated by simple adjustments of their home routines. For more involved symptoms she devised a method playing with the children in their home and simultaneously being available to the mother. This availability consisted initially of assisting a family in very concrete ways (for example, by helping them to obtain extra welfare benefits), demonstrating concern, and providing the mother with a feeling of self-worth. This, Fraiberg suggested, would in turn permit the mother to provide more satisfactorily for her infant's emotional development. Later reports of Fraiberg's work (1980) are more specific. Three types of intervention are described:

(1) Brief crisis intervention. This is used when the infant is in crisis, for example, when a parent has died or left the home or a sibling has arrived. The treatment consists of three to six meetings with the baby and mother during which the therapist may explain the baby's feelings. Simultaneously the therapist helps the parent to find appropriate alternate care if that is needed or provide her with some time for herself. The aim is to establish a new equilibrium within the family that will further the development of the infant and assist and support the family members in their caretaking roles.

(2) Developmental guidance. This treatment method is used where a parent has basically good abilities but the infant's physical or mental condition (blindness or infantile autism, for example) makes care difficult. Fraiberg states that it may also be the treatment of choice for parents whose infant is disturbed because of parental discord or other interpersonal conflict when parents seem unable to deal with internal conflicts.

During the actual session the therapist may demonstrate to a mother that the baby is crying because she is missing her and in this way reinforce the notion of the mother's importance to her infant. The therapist may also model how to talk to or feed this particular infant and by identification help the mother to improve her own interactions with this baby. The emphasis during all these therapeutic interactions remains on the infant who serves as a catalyst for the therapist's guidance and advice. While problems displayed by infants are often reflections of parental difficulties, the changes brought about by the birth of an infant will often force parents to reevaluate their own priorities and values and in this sense make them more open to developmental guidance. Fraiberg's own data suggest that the benefit from such an intervention can often be substantial.

(3) Infant-parent psychotherapy. This type of therapy will use selective material or conflicts of the caretaker, brought to light by the infant's behavior, and analyze their meaning or significance. The theoretic assumption is that an infant will often function as a transference object of his or her mother or father. Consequently, their relationship with him or her will reflect unresolved fears or traumata of the parents' past, which, in turn, will prevent them from providing appropriately for their infant. For example, a mother may perceive her infant as a "monster" who drains her and can never be satisfied. This may reflect the mother's own experience as a youngster, when taking and receiving was associated with stealing strength and energy from her parents and therefore had to be curbed so as not to hurt them. A baby who seemingly unashamedly seeks out food and comfort can, in such a scenario, easily be seen as a greedy monster stirring up hateful feelings in his or her mother. Likewise, a crying baby may represent a "lost" child who died two years ago and has not yet been sufficiently mourned. Such a mother, rather than seeking to understand the source of her infant's crying, may either become depressed herself and withdraw from the baby or get mad at him or her for "reminding her" of her previous loss.

Fraiberg will open up such isolated conflicts with a parent of her small patient but leave alone other problems that, while being equally serious, do not interfere with the present developmental needs of the infant. She will then literally make the connection between mother's past life experiences and present feelings and continue to work with such mothers for many months on a regular basis. However, each opening up of a conflictual area is accompanied by concrete supportive measures, and in this sense Fraiberg balances nurturance with the frequently painful self-scrutiny taking place in these families. It may in fact be this combination of concrete support, compassion, and explorative therapy that makes this form of psychotherapy appropriate for a wide range of parents, including teenage mothers and parents with serious psychiatric disorders.

Other clinicians have provided case examples where they were successful in assisting mothers in fostering or reestablishing a stable attachment with their infants (Escalona, 1945; Shapiro et al., 1976). However, there have also been reports of interventions leading to the adoption of an infant into a different home as changes in the parents could not be brought about (Ferholt & Provence, 1976).

Greenspan (1981) and his group at the National Institute of Mental Health, whose concepts of infant development and clinical assessment of infants have been discussed in earlier chapters, have developed specific treatment paradigms for infants and their families. Greenspan's interventions are developed from a detailed therapeutic diagnostic assessment of an infant and designed to assist in clearly identifiable areas of developmental delay or conflict. Thus an infant of 30 months may be helped in his or her attempts to achieve representational differentiation (to help the child comprehend that all 1-year-old children need help in walking) while a 20-month-old toddler may be stimulated in his or her ability to organize internal representation (to understand, for example, that mother always goes to work after breakfast). Many of Greenspan's actual treatment suggestions are similar to those of Fraiberg and Provence, but he especially stresses the use of the most developed segments of an infant's behavior as "a carrier" for helping an infant in his or her behavioral organization or any other developmental task. For example, a toddler may find it hard to show warmth or intimacy but is good at playing age-appropriate games. The therapist may play with this child in an especially warm manner, encouraging him to accept and use modifications in his interactions with others.

Parents are always active partners in Greenspan's treatment model. They are initially encouraged to observe themselves and their reactions to their infants. Later they may be asked to reflect how their conduct might contribute to their children's behavior. This then may finally help them to distinguish between issues related to their fantasy, mental imagery, and reality.

Symptomatic Behavioral Counseling

In contrast to such attempts to influence the parents' dynamic perception of their infant's needs, other clinicians have focused more on actual maternal behavior. For example, Sterba (1941) and Buxbaum (1947), who reported on infants from 8 to 20 months of age, simply instructed their mothers to change their handling of their infants. Although their advice was based on their own psychoanalytic conceptualization of the possible dynamic significance of each infant's symptoms, this was apparently not shared with the mothers.

Finally, Thomas and associates (1968), reporting from their longitudinal New York study, found that 3 of the 42 children in their clinical sample showed symptoms prior to 30 months of age. Treatment of these young children consisted exclusively of parent counseling. In fact, in all instances treatment sessions dealt with the "here and now" of the specific symptoms of each infant and usually lasted only two or three sessions. This "problem-oriented" approach by Chess and her group (1974) is undoubtedly practiced by many clinicians dealing with mildly or moderately troubled children and their families.

There are also numerous accounts of pediatricians and other health specialists who have become involved in parent counseling (see Augenbraun, 1967; Brazelton, 1962; Carey, 1968; Cullen, 1976). Since their treatment is usually of a more superficial nature and directed toward the parent only, we will not discuss it in this chapter. The same applies to infant stimulation programs. Such programs usually focus primarily on the cognitive aspects of an infant's development and rarely conceptualize the total needs of a child and his or her family (Ramey, 1982). Some aspects of this type of work undoubtedly incorporate principles of developmental guidance as outlined by Fraiberg (1980). However, stimulation programs do not deal with the inner life of an infant or his or her caretakers. We will likewise not review the accumulating evidence that suggests that specific day care or nursery programs may benefit deprived or socially disadvantaged infants or toddlers. Data pertaining to this literature can be found in a previous publication (Minde & Minde, 1981); but again, such programs, in our opinion, do not qualify as psychiatric treatment of infants. However, they should remind us that mental health professionals must be teamworkers who understand the contribution their colleagues in other disciplines can make to the care of an infant. As has been pointed out all through this book, an infant's life is made up of a variety of experiences. The mental health specialist whose training provides him or her with a good understanding of early development and the inner life of his or her patients and their caretakers and with pharmacological and medical treatment methods, is potentially well suited to take a leading role in the integration of broad-based treatment endeavors for infants and their families. The actual practical contribution of other professionals to the treatment of an infant may, nevertheless, be far more substantial. For example, a sensitive nursery school teacher is probably more important for the restitution of trust toward the world in a 2-year-old than a psychiatrist or psychologist can ever be.

Finally, we must temper our clinical impressions about the apparent efficacy of treatment in infancy with the sober awareness that there exists presently no scientifically acceptable study that has examined the effects of various types of counseling or therapy on infant and family growth and development. Yet we do know that up to 50% of the problems shown by 12- or 24-month-old infants are still present by the age of 4½ years and do not just disappear in the course of growing up (Jenkins et al., 1984). This suggests that we have a real need for effective intervention. The absence of studies in this area may discourage some clinicians from a therapeutic involvement with this age group. They may also serve as a challenge for us to provide such a data base for the benefit of both our colleagues and the children and their families who need our help in the future.

12

CASES THAT DO NOT FIT AND WHAT TO DO ABOUT THEM

In previous chapters we have discussed a number of conceptual issues related to infancy. We have also described the clinical picture, treatment, and prognosis of five specific disorders of infancy. Yet many parents or other professionals who consult infant mental health workers bring infants whose symptoms do not fit any of the five syndromes described. According to our experiences, they also want to consult us in a preventive manner, especially in the case of very young children with chronic or severe medical illnesses that appear to affect their present behavior. We are also frequently consulted by social workers and legal professionals in matters pertaining to custody or state wardship of infants. Since the educational and preventive aspects of infant psychiatry are important objectives to its practitioners, the present chapter will discuss, with the help of four cases, some of the questions and problems that have been posed to us by pediatricians as well as individual parents in hospitals and by social workers active in the courts and in adoption or child welfare agencies.

The discussion of these cases will replicate the infant mental health specialist's decision-making process, hence mentioning his or her hypotheses as well as actions. As all the case examples are based on actual clinical experiences, some progress notes on the families will also be given. In all instances identities as well as location and other identifying characteristics have been changed to preserve anonymity.

CONSULTATIONS TO MEDICAL INSTITUTIONS

There are basically two types of acute or chronic medical conditions where an infant mental health worker may be of assistance: those that are diagnosed soon after birth and keep an infant in hospital for a long time and conditions that require hospitalization later on during the early years resulting in behaviors that cause stress and anxiety in parents and staff.

Acute or Chronic Medical Conditions
Diagnosed Soon After Birth

The most common examples here are the premature birth of a baby with all the ensuing anxiety for the parents; children who require major medical interventions because of congenital abnormalities or chronic neonatal illness (for example, the tracheotomy for endotracheal stenosis or abdominal and thoracic surgery for a fistula between the esophagus and the trachea); and infants who suffer from a congenital disorder where normal or any survival may be questionable.

Such children are referred either because their parents or physicians are concerned about their abnormal development or because their parents are so severely stressed that they require special help and assistance. Other, more general issues confronting the clinician in such cases often center around the following questions:

(1) How much should parents of newborn infants visit their babies to "facilitate bonding"?
(2) How can parents be made to feel more like parents rather than visitors—especially when their baby is in the intensive care setting where most of the day-to-day decisions pertaining to this infant's life are made by a physician and routine care is provided by specially trained nurses?
(3) How much will the pain and discomfort experienced by many of these babies influence their later development and general outlook on life?
(4) How much is the general developmental delay so frequently observed in hospital-reared infants permanent or how can it best be remedied or prevented?

While the answers to these questions are complex and need to be tailored to the individual parent and infant, as a general response we would suggest that the following facilities and support systems should be available for infants who remain in hospital after birth for more than one month and for their families.

(1) Each intensive care nursery or infant ward should have facilities that make visiting for parents a comfortable task; for example, there should be rocking chairs, the opportunity for breast feeding or pumping, and facilities where parents can be alone with their infants.

(2) All professionals who work with infants should be carefully selected and provided with opportunities for regular in-service training. The physician who provides care to the infants should be identified to the parents and he or she should actively approach the parents and tell them of their infant's progress. Each unit of 20 beds should also have at least one full time social worker to provide support for the infants' families.

(3) Parents who have not visited their infant within two weeks after admission to an intensive care unit or an infant ward should be asked to come to a "formal" meeting with the physician in charge. This meeting can be set up with the primary aim of informing the parents about the medical status of their infant. After the meeting, both the physician and the parents can visit the baby together. During this visit the doctor or the nurse can explain the behavior and the condition of the baby in more detail. This method of bringing together parents and a small or ill infant is especially helpful with families who have come from countries where small, ill babies are unlikely to survive.

(4) Each hospitalized infant should have a primary nurse assigned to him or her for the total hospitalization. This nurse can monitor the parents' visiting patterns and will often be able to determine details of the family's personal and social background. This may give important clues about their parenting abilities and alert other professionals if additional support is needed.

(5) Parents should be given every opportunity to partake in the care of their hospitalized infants. There should be no limits to parental and sibling visits, and parents should be encouraged to get involved early in the routine infant care. Breast feeding should be encouraged. Such activities will allow the baby to become familiar with his or her parents and avoid potential difficulties in the parents' attachment to their baby (Minde, 1984).

(6) Parents of infants who have been in hospital a long time should have the opportunity to sleep one or two nights with their infants, in a room separate from the nursery, prior to the infant's discharge from hospital. This will familiarize the parents with the infant and will

diminish their fears associated with the infant's transfer from hospital to home.

(7) Parents whose infants have a chronic nonremediable disorder often need even more active support to develop a feeling that their infants have a life ahead of them. The feeling of "not knowing what is in store" and the frequent perception that these infants are "completely different from normal babies" often do not allow parents to conceptualize their proper role in the caretaking process and make them unsure in their dealings with these infants. An effective way to increase feelings of competence in such parents is through group meetings with other parents of similarly affected infants (Minde et al., 1980). Such meetings can be led by social workers or even parents who have gone through such an experience during the past year.

CASE EXAMPLE

Case 6

The director of a neonatal intensive care unit wanted assistance in the case of Mrs. M., a 35-year-old woman, an accomplished writer of children's books, who had given birth to her first child, named Marie, four weeks before. Both the pregnancy and delivery were medically uneventful but six hours after birth the newborn had a major epileptic seizure lasting for one hour. Investigations disclosed an absent right cerebral hemisphere. Both parents were informed about the diagnosis by the pediatrician. While the father seemed to take it philosophically, the mother said repeatedly that she wanted the baby to die and had not visited the infant since birth. The physician and nursery staff wanted advice on how to handle this situation.

Procedure of consultation. The infant mental health specialist initially informed himself about the rare medical condition so as to (1) assess the parents' factual knowledge of their infant's condition and place their feelings in some medical context and (2) learn more about the pediatrician's feelings about the disorder and the way he transmitted the diagnosis to the parents.

On talking with the pediatrician it became obvious that he had never seen an infant like this and hence had no personal experience with the future outlook for such children. However, he mentioned that recent tests had also found that the baby could not concentrate her urine, suggesting damage to the pituitary gland and the possibility of *diabetes insipidus*. He also mentioned that the textbook indicated little chance of survival for such an infant, but that he had not talked to the parents about this. This suggested that the pediatrician was himself somewhat uncertain about his future dealings with this family, which made it especially important to work closely with him.

The consultant spoke to Mrs. M. alone to learn more about her thoughts and feelings and her past life. This interview showed Mrs. M. to come from a solid family with many professional members. The commitment of her family to education had always been very high. She herself had never been ill, never seen a mental health professional, and had no history of panic attacks or irrational fears. She slept poorly— only four hours a night intermittently—and ate little but had not experienced any weight loss since the birth of the infant. She had thought of her baby a great deal but could at times be distracted from such thoughts when watching a television show or being engaged in a conversation. She also stressed that she did not want to talk about the baby to others but wished that she could do so with her husband. He, however, seemed not keen to do so and hence the future of the infant had not been discussed between them.

During the interview her fears centered around the fact that she would not be able to carry on writing books as all her time would have to be spent with her disabled girl. She also mentioned how she was afraid to visit Maria as she might then "begin to love her" and end up looking after her, hating herself at the same time for having forsaken her career. Mrs. M. cried a few times during the interview but said that this was the first time she had done so since the baby was born.

The consultant then spoke to the father alone to assess his background, present feelings for his wife and his infant, and the effect the crisis had on him. Mr. M. presented as a 43-year-old lawyer who came from a poor Catholic family. He had worked very hard to achieve his present status and had given up many things that were important to him during his childhood to do so. Thus he did not attend church any more and did not keep close contact with his four siblings. He had married his wife five years ago as he "felt ready to start such a union" and had enjoyed their culturally rich life. He had been somewhat ambivalent about his wife's wish to have a baby and had not yet decided how serious the infant's condition really was. However, he was prepared to go along with any plan that would be acceptable to his wife, although he had not yet discussed this with her.

The father had shown no changes in his sleeping, eating, or working patterns and had also supported his wife's decision to go away for three days alone to their cottage to finish a children's book she had to deliver to her publishers soon. He had interpreted this as a "sign of progress." The mother's aging parents and her sister had not been actively involved with her after the baby's birth, but many of her colleagues and friends had shown sincere sympathy. The available information suggested that the M.s' marriage was based on companionship and common experiences but that in a time of crisis, both parents had a tendency to deal with issues in their own way.

Finally, the consultant spent some time with Maria, who at 6 weeks weighed 10½ pounds and was still in an isolette in the hospital. Maria was a moderately attractive baby who had blond hair but an obvious left-sided spastic paralysis and did not focus visually (she was in fact officially diagnosed to be blind one week later). However, she moulded well with the caretaker and cried when she was put back into her incubator and left by herself. Hence she responded quickly to being touched and held and obviously had good hearing. Because of an associated large cleft palate Maria was very difficult to feed but, according to nurses' notes, slept up to six hours during the night although she was considered to be an "unhappy baby" by the nursing staff.

Summary and recommendations. In summary, the M.s were seen as basically competent parents who had a primarily intellectually comforting union. Both partners were very engrossed in their individual work and seemed not prepared to make major changes in their lives for Maria when forced to do so. The father did not provide the mother with much emotional support and seemed basically more reserved with the infant than was the mother. The mother also did not seem to wish to change her relationship with her husband but looked for concrete guidance and advice on whether she should institutionalize Maria or take her home and give up her career.

To provide both parents with some concrete information, the pediatrician and the mental health consultant saw them both together. Initially they discussed the positive and negative aspects of Maria's illness but stressed there was a wide range of services available to both Maria and them. For example, they emphasized that if the M.s placed their infant, others would provide good care for her and like her. They also discussed various other possible arrangements, from a full day care program to a twice-weekly day placement in an infant group. The message here was that the parents could choose from a spectrum of services, giving various degrees of involvement.

This approach reassured mother that her mixed feelings about the infant were respected and "normal." Her anxiety decreased markedly and after some four weeks she did take Maria home and with some outside help managed well for seven months, at which time the baby died.

**Infants Hospitalized During
the First Four Years of Life**

It has been demonstrated in a number of studies (Douglas, 1975; Quinton & Rutter, 1976) that children who are hospitalized between the ages of 6 and 48 months show a significantly higher incidence of emotional and conduct disorders later in life. These disturbances are independent of other family problems although children who come from problem families are more likely to suffer from long-term adverse effects of the hospitalization than do children from well-adjusted families.

The acute symptoms shown by hospitalized infants are

(1) increased irritability and decreased frustration tolerance,
(2) withdrawal and depressive reactions,
(3) regression to an earlier developmental level, and
(4) increased behavioral problems, especially of an oppositional nature (Prugh & Eckhard, 1980).

Other factors that influence an infant's reaction to hospitalization are the length and frequency of the stay in hospital (Mrazek, 1984), the ability of the parents to be with their infant in hospital (Ferguson, 1979), and the characteristics of the institution. Thus, hospitalized young children need sensitive staff who are consistently available, will prepare the children for specific procedures, and will allow appropriate and consistent stimulation and activity (Mrazek, 1984).

Parents obviously play a crucial part in this system as they can provide much of the continuity of care so important for the development of an infant. However, it is important to realize that parents also need support. While such support usually translates into an active partnership between medical staff and the parents, at times such support may also mean that a nurse or physician suggests that mother or father take a break away from their baby and have a night at home, so as to get away from the hospital routine.

CASE EXAMPLE

Case 7

Ms. N., an 18-year-old single high school student, and the mother of 3-month-old Nicholas, was referred to a psychiatrist by the nursing staff of the surgical ward where Nicholas had lived since birth, to obtain advice on how to get mother more involved in the day-to-day care of Nicholas. Allegedly Ms. N. came only twice a week to see Nicholas and even then rarely stayed more than 45 minutes. During these visits she was reported to look at and stroke Nicholas rather perfunctorily, but had refused to feed him or even change one diaper. Nicholas had been born with a fistula between his esophagus and trachea. His abnormality had been diagnosed soon after his birth as he spat and coughed up all his food, which led to his transfer from a general hospital to a pediatric infancy ward.

The mother, who had been interviewed before by a social worker, was the oldest of three children of a working-class family. Her father had immigrated from Europe 21 years ago and was seen as a strict disciplinarian who had not allowed his daughter to go out on dates until she was 16 years old. Her illegitimate pregnancy had been a major blow to him, and he had not talked to his daughter until about six weeks before Nicholas's birth. Her mother had never worked and was allegedly quite happy to raise Nicholas as her fourth child. She had in fact visited the boy more than had his mother and had suggested to some nurses that her daughter surely was not fit to be a mother yet.

Nicholas's father, Bill K., was a 20-year-old laborer who lived at home and who was interested in his baby and in Ms. N. He worked regularly on a construction job but came to visit Nicholas alone quite regularly, had changed his diapers on several occasions, and seemed quite keen to take him home.

Nicholas, meanwhile, had been placed on his back right after admission with both his hands tied to the mattress to prevent him from sucking his thumb and by doing so increase his production of saliva. He was fed through a gastrostomy tube directly into his stomach and had a nasogastric tube that constantly suctioned away the saliva he produced in his mouth. As he had to remain in this fixed position all the time, he had never been on his stomach, tasted food or his thumb, and had never been carried around by anyone.

However, ten days before the consultation, Nicholas's fistula had been closed surgically. This now allowed him to be lifted off his bed, be carried around, and see the gradual institution of regular oral feedings. The medical staff was greatly concerned, however, that his mother's unwillingness to participate in Nicholas's care at that time would compromise his later development.

In an attempt to assess the parents' understanding of the situation, they were both asked to come for an interview together. Ms. N. brought Nicholas along to the first interview and while we were not sure whether this meant that mother wanted to "hide" behind her baby, we quickly realized that we were participating in a very special demonstration of maternal concern. Thus the mother quickly began to talk about her mother's interference with her attempts to be a mother to Nicholas and how she was made to feel so incompetent that she hardly dared to touch the boy. In fact, the mother's understanding of Nicholas's needs was far more appropriate than anyone had thought possible (she insisted on keeping Nicholas on her lap during our initial talk rather than in his pram since "he now needed lots of body contact").

Summary and recommendations. In summary Ms. N. and Bill K. were young but interested parents whose struggle against their own needs for dependency confounded their freedom to parent Nicholas. While neither Ms. N. nor Bill seemed to be able to look after Nicholas on their own at that time, we felt that they had to be given a gradually increasing range of parenting tasks. At the same time we hoped to replace some of the support Ms. N. got from her own mother, which was often associated with scoldings and humiliation, by shifting it to the occupational therapist who we hoped would provide more peer support. Therefore, we initially set up some regular times during which Nicholas's father would visit Ms. N. at her home and have them "both" look after "their baby."

Later interviews in the hospital included the occupational therapist who advised on toys and other environmental stimulation for Nicholas. The boy, who had functioned at a 2-week level in his general motor and social behavior when he was seen initially, in fact quickly rallied and four weeks later functioned at an 8- to 10-week developmental level.

Despite this initial success, things did not continue to go smoothly as Nicholas was readmitted to hospital three more times during the ensuing six months because he had lost weight and would not feed enough.

While the surgeons were sure that his feeding difficulties were due to his initial fistula and operation, Nicholas's episodes of vomiting were always precipitated by arguments between Nicholas's mother and her own mother. These setbacks notwithstanding, Nicholas did catch up in his milestones and at 1 year seemed eager to grow and develop.

CONSULTATIONS TO LEGAL OR CHILD WELFARE AGENCIES

Another group of cases brought to an infant psychiatrist involves

(1) children whose parents show difficulties of a nature that requires the state to step in to protect the child, and
(2) children whose parents have difficulties in their relationship with each other and want guidance on how best to handle the development of their child in such a situation.

While most legal and welfare cases are complex and differ from each other in important ways, the following vignettes give at least some ideas of the range of problems facing an infant psychiatrist.

CASE EXAMPLES

Case 8

Ms. O., an 18-year-old unmarried mother of a 9-month old baby, contacted a local welfare agency with the wish to place her infant for three to four months to give her time to "decide what to do with her life." The welfare worker arranged for a consultation with an infant mental health specialist to see how this request could be handled without jeopardizing the infant's long-term relationship with his mother.

The aims of our initial interview with Ms. O. were

(1) to assess the mother's personal strengths and weaknesses: thus we wanted to know about the relationships she had had with adults during her childhood as well as her past and present learning and occupational history;
(2) to learn something about that mother's motivation for placing her son John—was it a repeating pattern of disengaging herself whenever she was

required to make a commitment or did she indeed require some time out to work on some more basic issues? Did she need to cope with angry feelings toward John?—this we hoped to do by assessing the quality of her previous relationship with John and her support system.

The interview revealed that Ms. O. had been raised in a poor family, the second of four children. Her father did not have regular work and physically abused her mother but left when Ms. O. was 9 years old. Her mother had worked in the kitchen of a hospital. She had been very strict and punitive with her four children and never had time to play with them. Ms. O. finished ninth grade but left home at 16 and has had virtually no contact with her family since then. However, there was an aunt who had taken her in at that time and who was also with her during the delivery of John. This lady had seven children of her own and while she minded Ms. O.'s infant on a number of occasions, she did not want to raise the infant. Ms. O. had not seen the father of John since he left town six months ago. He provided her with no child support.

Ms. O. who had never worked for more than 2 months at any one job, hoped to travel through North America by herself once the baby was placed. She then wanted to finish high school and "get a good job." Ms. O. had not been in trouble with the law and did not abuse drugs or alcohol.

John was seen with his mother at the agency a week later when he was 9½ months old. He weighed 19 pounds and looked healthy. He sat well and could pivot easily, but was not easily engaged in any activity because of his apparent need to hold on to his mother. However, once his mother agreed to keep him on her lap, he became more focused in his behavior. For example, he took a cube in each hand and bumped them together. He also picked up a pellet with a good radial grasp and did make some babbling noises. He played with his toes and once even put them in his mouth. However, he did not imitate the examiner tapping the table, never crawled away from his mother to explore the room (even though he was reported to do so at home), and would not release a cube into a cup. He also did not hand anything to his mother and did not smile at her. Ms. O. in turn showed little delight in her infant but administered to him appropriately. She did not talk much to John and did not encourage him to pursue a particular activity.

This interview indicated that John had good basic abilities but showed a number of symptoms compatible with inconsistent caretaking (such as his lack of smiling, exploration, and imitation). On further questioning his mother did admit that John had been left with a number of her friends for one or two days all through his life and that he would often sleep poorly and would be especially clingy after such visits.

Summary and recommendations. John's mother appeared to have had a moderately unstable childhood and comparatively few long-standing positive interpersonal relationships. Her wish to see the world was possibly an attempt to make up for her deprivation. As she had neither funds nor people to go to, the likelihood of this plan succeeding without complications and further damage to her precarious self-esteem was not high. That also made it unlikely that she would be able to provide well for John for some time to come without substantial outside support.

The initial plan was to have the agency offer Ms. O. substitute care for John (such as a good day care program) and education and stimulation for herself (through schooling for adults combined with group sessions on life-management skills with other parents in a similar situation). This plan was rejected, indicating Ms. O.'s fear of "the establishment" and her mistrust of the intentions of the agency.

The next plan was to place John in a home that could keep him for a long time if that proved necessary, to set up regular visiting times for mother to maintain some ties between them, and to provide Ms. O. with an invitation to join the programs mentioned above. The aim here was to prevent John from experiencing more than one placement and give his mother the option of establishing or reestablishing contact with him when she felt psychologically ready for it.

The mother accepted this plan, left town shortly afterward, and has not recontacted the agency for 14 months. She did telephone John's foster family on four occasions but was vague as to her exact whereabouts and future plans. John has adapted well to his foster parents and at 24 months called them mama and papa.

Case 9

Mr. P., a 35-year-old lawyer, had asked his lawyer to contact an infant psychiatrist to help him regain custody of his 2½-year-old son Brian. His physician wife had left him nine months ago and had been awarded custody of Brian. Mr. P. felt that the boy now needed a father more urgently than a mother to establish his "sexual identity." He felt that a psychiatrist would support him in this "developmental demand."

As a mental health professional's primary aim is to support the best interest of the infant, it seemed important to learn more about the parents' previous relationship and their present feelings for each other.

Mr. P. initially refused to meet the psychiatrist directly, preferring to have his lawyer speak for him. After some hesitation, however, he did come, and indicated that he had helped his wife a great deal financially during their marriage, which coincided with her later student and early internship years. He also stated that he was still severely hurt by her sudden departure with a younger physician colleague. He himself had always preferred a regulated life and had been unable to match his wife's more extroverted lifestyle.

Asked about his plans for Brian, Mr. P. hoped to place his son in a good day care center and felt comfortable in looking after him by himself. At present, visiting arrangements gave him access to Brian each Saturday afternoon and Sunday and alternate Wednesday evenings and nights. Mr. P. felt that his son Brian enjoyed his days with him and would like to live with him all the time although he had never directly said so.

In the struggle between parents for an infant it is generally helpful to assess both parents and the infant. However, the other parent is legally not required to appear for an interview and the appointment with him or her in fact is best arranged by the accusing party, leaving the mental health professional outside the personal struggle of the parents. It should also be stressed to both parties that the infant psychiatrist would share his or her evaluation of the present caretaking environment amongst all parties and that he or she cannot enforce changes in the present custody arrangement. These can only be mandated by a court of law.

In Mr. P.'s case, his estranged wife did agree to meet the psychiatrist but did not want to bring her son along as she did not want him to be confused by the parental struggle. Mrs. P. presented as a 29-year-old woman who had just finished her third year of residency. She had moved in with her new companion nine months ago, together with Brian, and claimed that this move had benefited the boy. While previously the arguments with her husband caused so much tension in the house that Brian would sleep poorly and cry a lot, he now was a happy, outgoing youngster who ate well, talked a blue streak, and seemed to show no psychological difficulties. As he had remained in his previous day care program where he liked the staff, mother saw no need to change the present arrangement. Mother also felt that Brian was very much aware of being a boy—he was fascinated with certain male singing stars on television, played the father in most family games, and enjoyed a wide variety of toys usually preferred by boys. He also allegedly liked his visits with his father but always seemed glad to be home with mother again.

Summary and conclusions. The mental health specialist is frequently drawn into private disputes of parents who, by using developmental slogans such as "sexual identity" or "separation crisis," try to work out their personal conflicts. In general, he or she will attempt to refocus the parents' feelings on the marital partners and in this way help them to work through their personal concerns. The diversity of human nature makes it extremely difficult to judge the specific appropriateness of a mother or father in helping the child achieve a new developmental stage. It is, therefore, clearly in the best interest of the child to remain neutral in such situations.

REFERENCES

Affleck, G., Tennen, H., & Gershman, K. (1984, April). *Initial validation of an attribution-control analysis of maternal coping with newborn intensive care.* Presented at the Fourth Biennial International Conference on Infant Studies, New York.

Ainsworth, M., Blehar, M., Waters, E., & Walls, S. (1978). *Patterns of attachment.* Hillsdale, NJ: Erlbaum.

Alpern, G. D., Boll, T. J., & Shearer, M. S. (1980). *Developmental profile II.* Aspen, CO: Psychological Development Publications.

Alpert, A. (1959). Reversibility of pathological fixations associated with maternal deprivation in infancy. *Psychoanalytic Study of the Child, 14,* 169-185.

Alpert, A. (1967). Prenursery project: Indications and counter-indications for therapeutic intervention in the prenursery via the mother. *Psychoanalytic Study of the Child, 22,* 139-155.

Alpert, A., Neubauer, P. B., & Weil, A. (1956). Unusual variations in drive endowment. *Psychoanalytic Study of the Child, 11,* 125-163.

Als, H. (1982). Towards a synactive theory of development: Promise for the assessment and support of infant individuality. *Infant Mental Health Journal, 3,* 229-243.

Als, H., & Brazelton, T. B. (1981). A new model of assessing the behavioral organization in preterm and fullterm infants. *Journal of the American Academy of Child Psychiatry, 20,* 239-263.

Als, H., Lester, B. M., Tronick, E. C., & Brazelton, T. B. (1982a). Toward a research instrument for the assessment of preterm infants' behavior (APIB). In H. E. Fitzgerald, B. M. Lester, & M. W. Yogman (Eds.), *Theory and research in behavioral pediatrics* (Vol. 1). New York: Plenum.

Als, H., Lester, B. M., Tronick, E. C., & Brazelton, T. B. (1982b). Manual for the assessment of preterm infants' behavior (APIB). In H. E. Fitzgerald, B. M. Lester, & M. W. Yogman (Eds.), *Theory and research in behavioral pediatrics* (Vol. 1). New York: Plenum.

Als, H., Tronick, E., Lester, B. M., & Brazelton, T. B. (1979). Specific neonatal measures: The Brazelton Neonatal Behavioral Assessment Scale. In J. D. Osovsky (Ed.), *Handbook of infant development.* New York: Wiley.

Amsterdam, B. K. (1972). Mirror self-image reactions before age 2. *Developmental Psychology, 5,* 297-305.

Anders, T. (1974). The infant sleep profile. *Neuropaediatrie, 5,* 425-442.

Anders, T. (1978). Home-recorded sleep in two- and nine-month-old infants. *Journal of the Academy of Child Psychiatry, 17,* 421-432.

Anders, T. (1982). A longitudinal study of night time sleep-wake patterns in infants from birth to one year. In J. D. Call & E. Galenson (Eds.), *Frontiers of infant psychiatry.* New York: Basic Books.

Anders, T., & Sostek, A. (1976). The use of time lapse video recording of sleep-wake behavior in human infants. *Psychophysiology, 13,* 155-158.

Anders, T., & Weinstein, P. (1972). Sleep and its disorders in infants and children: A review. *Pediatrics, 50,* 312-324.

Andronico, M. P., Fidler, J., Guerney, B. G., & Guerney, L. (1967). The combination of didactic and dynamic elements in filial therapy. *International Journal of Group Therapy, 17*, 10-17.

Arend, R., Gove, F. L., & Sroufe, L. A. (1979). Continuity of individual adaptation from infancy to kindergarten: A predictive study of ego-resiliency and curiosity in pre-schoolers. *Child Development, 50*, 950-959.

Ariès, P. (1962). *Centuries of childhood. A social history of family life.* New York: Knopf.

Aserinsky, E., & Kleitman, N. (1953). Regularly occurring periods of eye motility and concomitant phenomena during sleep. *Science, 118*, 273-274.

Auerbach, A. B. (1968). *Parents learn through discussion.* New York: Wiley.

Augenbraun, B., Reid, H., & Friedman, D. (1967). Brief intervention as a preventive force in disorders of early childhood. *American Journal of Orthopsychiatry, 37*, 697-702.

Baer, D. M. (1970). An age-irrelevant concept of development. *Merrill-Palmer Quarterly, 16*, 238-245.

Baltes, P. B., Reese, H. W., & Lipsitt, L. P. (1980). Life-span developmental psychology. *Annual Review of Psychology, 31*, 65-100.

Bandura, A. (1977). Toward a unifying theory of behavioral change. *Psychological Review, 84*, 191-215.

Bangs, T. E., & Dodson, S. (1979). *Birth to three: Developmental scale.* Hingham, MA: Teaching Resources.

Barbero, G. J., & Shaheen, E. (1967). Environmental failure to thrive: A clinical view. *Journal of Pediatrics, 71*, 639-644.

Bayley, N. (1969). *Bayley scales of infant development: Birth to two years.* New York: Psychological Corporation.

Beery, K. (1967). *Developmental test of visual motor integration.* Chicago: Follett.

Bell, S. M., & Ainsworth, M.D.S. (1972). Infant crying and maternal responsiveness. *Child Development, 43*, 1171-1190.

Belsky, J. (Ed.). (1981). *In the beginning: Readings in infancy.* New York: Columbia University Press.

Bentler, P. M. (1962). An infant's phobia treated with reciprocal inhibition therapy. *Journal of Child Psychology and Psychiatry, 3, 185-189.*

Bergman, P., & Escalona, S. K. (1949). Unusual sensitivities in very young children. *Psychoanalytic Study of the Child, 3/4*, 333-352.

Berkowitz, P. B., & Graziano, A. M. (1972). Training parents as behavior therapists: A review. *Behavior Research Therapy, 10*, 297-317.

Bernal, J. (1973). Night waking in infants during the first 14 months. *Developmental Medical Child Neurology, 14,* 362-372.

Bertalanffy, L. von (1968). *General system theory.* New York: Braziller.

Bettelheim, B. (1967). *The empty fortress: Infantile autism and the birth of the self.* New York: Free Press.

Birch, H. G., & Gussow, J. D. (1970). *Disadvantaged children: Health, nutrition, and school failure.* New York: Harcourt, Brace & World.

Belhar, M. (1974). Anxious attachment and defensive reactions associated with day care. *Child Development, 45*, 683-692.

Blurton-Jones, N., Rossetti Ferreira, M. C., Farquar Brown, M., & MacDonald, L. (1978). The association between perinatal factors and late night waking. *Developmental Medicine and Child Neurology, 20*, 427-434.

Bornstein, B. (1935). Phobia in a two-and-a-half-year-old child. *Psychoanalytic Quarterly, 4*, 93-119.

Bowlby, J. (1944). Fourty-four juvenile thieves: Their characters and home life. *International Journal of Psycho-Analysis, 25*, 19-52, 107-127.

Bowlby, J. (1951). Maternal care and mental health. *World Health Organization Monograph, No. 2.* London: Her Majesty's Stationery Office.

Bowlby, J. (1969). *Attachment and loss: I. Attachment.* New York: Basic Books.

Bowlby, J. (1973). *Attachment and loss: II. Separation, anxiety and anger.* London: Hogarth Press.

Bowlby, J. (1980). *Attachment and loss: III. Loss, sadness and depression.* New York: Basic Books.

Bowlby, J. (1982). *Attachment and loss II. Attachment* (2nd ed.). New York: Basic Books.

Bowlby, J. (1984). Violence in the family as a disorder of the attachment and caregiving systems. *American Journal of Psychoanalysis, 44,* 9-27.

Bowlby, J., Robertson, J., & Rosenbluth, D. (1952). A two-year-old goes to hospital. *Psychoanalytic Study of the Child, 7,* 82-94.

Brant, S., & Cullman, E. (1980). *Small folk: A celebration of childhood in America.* New York: Dutton.

Brazelton, T. B. (1962). A child-oriented approach to toilet-training. *Pediatrics, 29,* 121-128.

Brazelton, T. B. (1973). *Neonatal behavioral assessment scale.* Clinics in Developmental Medicine, No. 50. Philadelphia: Lippincott.

Brazelton, T. B., & Als, H. (1979). Four early stages in the development of mother-infant interaction. *Psychoanalytic Study of the Child, 34,* 349-369.

Brazelton, T. B., Koslowski, B., & Main, M. (1974). The origins of reciprocity. In M. Lewis & L. A. Rosenblum (Eds.), *The effect of the infant on its caregivers.* New York: Wiley.

Brazelton, T. B., Tronick, E., Adamson, L., Als, H., & Wise, S. (1975). Early mother-infant reciprocity. In M. A. Hofer (Ed.), *Parent-infant interaction.* London: CIBA.

Brazelton, T. B., Yogman, M. W., Als, H., & Tronick, E. (1979). The infant as a focus of family reciprocity. In M. Lewis & L. A. Rosenblum (Eds.), *The child and its family.* New York: Plenum Press.

Bretherton, I. (1980). Young children in stressful situations: The supporting role of attachment figures and unfamiliar caregivers. In G. V. Coelho & P. J. Ahmen (Eds.), *Uprooting and development.* New York: Plenum Press.

Brigance, A. H. (1978). *Brigance diagnostic inventory of early development.* North Billerica, MA: Curriculum Associates.

Brooks, J., & Weinraub, M. (1976). A history of infant intelligence testing. In M. Lewis (Ed.), *Origins of intelligence.* New York: Plenum Press.

Brown, G. W., & Rutter, M. (1966). The measurement of family activities and relationships—A methodological study. *Human Relations, 19,* 241-263.

Bruner, J. (1978). How to do things with words. In J. Bruner & A. Garton (Eds.), *Human growth and development.* Oxford: Oxford University Press.

Bruner, J., & Sherwood, V. (1976). Peek-a-boo and the learning of new structures. In J. Bruner, A. Jolly, & K. Silva (Eds.), *Play: Its role in evolution and development.* Harmondsworth: Penguin.

Bryen, D. N., & Gallagher, D. (1983). Assessment of language and communication. In K. D. Paget & B. A. Bracken (Eds.), *The psychoeducational assessment of preschool children.* New York: Grune & Stratton.

Burke, W. T., & Abidin, R. R. (1978). *The development of a parenting stress index.* Paper presented to the American Psychological Association.

Burlingham, D., & Freud, A. (1943). *Infants without families.* London: Allen & Unwin.

Buxbaum, E. (1947). Activity and aggression in children. *American Journal of Orthopsychiatry, 17,* 161-166.

Bzoch, K. R., & League, R. (1971). *The Bzoch-League receptive-expressive emergent language scale.* Gainesville, FL: Tree of Life Press.

Caldwell, B. M., & Bradley, R. H. (1979). *Home observation for measurement of the environment*. Little Rock: University of Arkansas Press.

Call, J. D. (1980). Attachment disorders of infancy. In H. I. Kaplan et al. (Eds.), *Comprehensive textbook of psychiatry* (3rd ed.). Baltimore, MD: Williams & Wilkins.

Campbell, M. (1976). Pharmacotherapy. In M. Rutter & E. Schopler (Eds.), *Autism: A reappraisal of concepts of treatment*. New York: Plenum Press.

Carew, J. V. (1980). Experience and the development of intelligence in young children at home and in day care. *Monographs of the Society for Research in Child Development*, *45* (6-7, Serial No. 187).

Carey, W. B. (1968). Maternal anxiety and infantile colic. Is there a relationship? *Clinical Pediatrics*, *7*, 590-595.

Carey, W. B. (1970). A simplified method for measuring infant temperament. *Journal of Pediatrics. 77*, 188-194.

Carey, W. B., & McDevitt, S. C. (1978). Revision of the infant temperament questionnaire. *Pediatrics*, *61*, 735-739.

Cattell, P. (1940). *Infant intelligence scale*. New York: Psychological Corporation.

Caulfield, E. (1931). *The infant welfare movement in the eighteenth century*. New York: Hoeber.

Chen, H., & Woolley, P. (1978). A developmental assessment chart for noninstitutionalized Down's-syndrome children. *Growth*, *42*, 157-165.

Chess, S. (1971). Autism in children with congenital rubella. *Journal of Autism and Childhood Schizophrenia*, *1*, 33-47.

Chess, S., Fernandez, P., & Korn, S. (1974). Behavioral consequences of congenital rubella. *Journal of Pediatrics*, *93*, 699-705.

Clark, P., & Rutter, M. (1981). Autistic children's responses to structure and to interpersonal demands. *Journal of Autism and Developmental Disorders*, *11*, 201-217.

Clarke-Stewart, K. A. (1973). Interactions between mothers and their young children: Characteristics and consequences. *Monographs of the Society for Research in Child Development, No. 38*. Chicago: University of Chicago Press.

Cohen, D. J., Caparulo, B. K., Gold, J. R., Waldo, M. C., Shaywit, B. A., Ruttenburg, B. A., & Rimland, B. (1978). Agreement in diagnosis: Clinical assessment and behavior rating scales for pervasively disturbed children. *Journal of the American Academy of Child Psychiatry, 17*, 689-703.

Cohen, R. L. (1979). The approach to assessment. In J. D. Call (Ed.), *Basic handbook of child psychiatry* (Vol. 1). New York: Basic Books.

Coons, C. E., Frankenburg, W. K., Garrett, C. J., Headley, R., & Fandal, A. W. (1978). Home screening questionnaire (HSQ). In W. D. Frankenburg (Ed.), *Proceedings of the Second International Conference on Developmental Screening*. Denver, CO: University of Colorado Press.

Cox, A., Hopkinson, K., & Rutter, M. (1981). Psychiatric interviewing techniques II. Naturalistic study: Eliciting factual information. *British Journal of Psychiatry, 138*, 283-291.

Cullen, K. J. (1976). A six-year controlled trial of prevention of children's behavior disorders. *Journal of Pediatrics, 88*, 662-666.

Damarin, F. (1978). Bayley scales of infant development. In O. K. Buros (Ed.), *The eighth mental measurements yearbook* (Vol. 1). Highland Park, NJ: Gryphon Press.

Darwin, C. R. (1877). Biographical sketch of an infant. *Mind, 7*.

Decarie, T. D. (1969). A study of the mental and emotional development of the thalidomide child. In B. M. Foss (Ed.), *Determinants of infant behavior* (Vol. 4). London: Methuen.

DeCasper, A. J., & Fifer, W. P. (1980). Of human bonding: newborns prefer their mothers' voices. *Science, 208 (4448)*, 1174-1176.

de Mause, L. (1974). *The history of childhood*. New York: Psychohistory Press.

deMyer, M., Barton, S., Alpern, G., Kimberlin, C., Allen, J., Yang, E., & Steele, R. (1974). The measured intelligence of autistic children. *Journal of Autism and Childhood Schizophrenia, 4*, 42-60.

deMyer, M. D., Hingtgen, J. N., & Jackson, R. K. (1981). Infantile autism reviewed: A decade of research. *Schizophrenia Bulletin, 7*, 388-395.

Dennis, M. (1984). Neuropsychological assessment since 1979. In J. Noshpitz, I. Berlin, J. Call, R. Cohen, S. Harrison, & L. Stone (Eds.), *Basic handbook of child psychiatry* (Vol. 5). New York: Basic Books.

de Sanctis, S. (1925). *Neuropsichiatria infantile*. Rome: Stock.

Deutsch, M. (1964). Facilitating development in the pre-school child: Social and psychological perspectives. *Merrill-Palmer Quarterly, 10*, 249-263.

Dewhurst, K. (1963). *John Locke (1632-1704). Physician and philosopher. A medical biography*. London: Wellcome Historical Medical Library.

Douglas, J.W.B. (1975). Early hospital admissions and later disturbances of behaviour and learning. *Developmental Medicine and Child Neurology, 17*, 456-480.

Drotar, D. (in press). Failure to thrive. In D. K. Routh (Ed.), *Handbook of pediatric psychology*. New York: Guilford.

DSM-III. (1980). *Diagnostic and statistical manual of mental disorders* (3rd ed.). Washington, DC: American Psychiatric Association.

Dunn, L. M. (1965). *Peabody picture vocabulary test*. Circle Pines, MN: American Guidance Service.

Dunn, L. M., & Dunn, L. M. (1981). *Peabody picture vocabulary test—Revised*. Circle Pines, MN: American Guidance Service.

Dunn, P. P. (1974). "That enemy is the baby": Childhood in imperial Russia. In L. de Mause (Ed.), *The history of childhood*. New York: Psychohistory Press.

Egan, J., Chatoor, I., & Rosen, G. (1980). Nonorganic failure to thrive: Pathogenesis and classification. *Clinical Proceedings of the Children's Hospital National Medical Center, 34*, 173-182.

Eisenberg, L., & Kanner, L. (1956). Early infantile autism: 1943-55. *American Journal of Orthopsychiatry, 26*, 556-566.

Emde, R. N., Gaensbauer, T. J., & Harmon, R. J. (1976). Emotional expression in infancy. A biobehavioral study. *Psychological Issues, 10*, Whole No. 37.

Emde, R. N., & Metcalf, D. (1970). An electroencephalographic study of behavioral rapid eye movement states in the human newborn. *Journal of Nervous and Mental Disease, 150*, 376-386.

Emde, R. N., & Robinson, J. (1979). The first 2 months: Recent research in developmental psychobiology. In J. D. Call, J. D. Noshpitz, R. C. Cohen, & I. N. Berlin (Eds.), *Basic handbook of child psychiatry*. New York: Basic Books.

Emmerich, W. (1968). Personality development and concepts of structure. *Child Development, 39*, 671-690.

English, P. (1984). Pediatrics and the unwanted child in history: Foundling homes, disease, and the origins of foster care in New York City, 1860 to 1920. *Pediatrics, 73*, 699-711.

Erickson, M. F., Sroufe, L. A., & Egeland, B. (1985). The relationship between quality of attachment and behavior problems in preschool in a high-risk sample. In I. Bretherton & E. Waters (Eds.), *Monographs Society for Research in Child Development, 50*(1-2, Serial No. 209).

Erikson, E. (1959). *Identity and the life cycle*. New York: Norton.

Erikson, E. (1963). *Childhood and society.* New York: Norton.

Escalona, S. K. (1945). Feeding disturbances in very young children. *American Journal of Orthopsychiatry, 15,* 76-80.

Escalona, S. K. (1962). The study of individual differences and the problem of state. *Journal of the American Academy of Child Psychiatry, 1,* 11-37.

Esman, A. H. (1983). The "stimulus barrier": A review and reconsideration. *Psychoanalytic Study of the Child, 38,* 193-207.

Fagan, J. F., & McGrath, S. K. (1981). Infant recognition memory and later intelligence. *Intelligence, 5,* 121-130.

Fantz, R. L., & Nevis, S. (1967). Pattern preferences and perceptual-cognitive development in early infancy. *Merrill-Palmer Quarterly, 13,* 77-108.

Ferguson, B. F. (1979). Preparing young children for hospitalizaiton. *Pediatrics, 64,* 656-664.

Ferholt, J., & Provence, S. (1976). Diagnosis and treatment of an infant with psychological vomiting. *The Psychoanalytic Study of the Child, 31,* 439-459.

Field, T. M. (1977). Effects of early separation, interactive deficit, and experimental manipulations on infant-mother face-to-face interaction. *Child Development, 48,* 763-771.

Field, T. M. (1982). Infants born at risk: Early compensatory experiences. In L. A. Bond & J. M. Joffe (Eds.), *Facilitating infant and early development.* Hanover: University Press of New England.

Fish, B., Campbell, M., & Wile, R. (1968). A classification of schizophrenic children under five years. *American Journal of Psychiatry, 124,* 1415-1423.

Fitzhardinge, P. (1985). Follow-up studies on small for dates infants. In M. Winick (Ed.), *Feeding the mother and infant.* New York: Wiley.

Fitzhardinge, P. M., & Stevens, E. M. (1974). The small for date infant. I. Later growth patterns. *Pediatrics, 49,* 671-681.

Folstein, S., & Rutter, M. (1977). Infantile autism: A genetic study of 21 twin pairs. *Journal of Child Psychology and Psychiatry, 18,* 297-321.

Forsyth, B.W.C., Leventhal, J. M., & McCarthy, P. L. (in press). Mothers' perceptions of problems of feeding and crying behaviors: A prospective study. *Pediatrics.*

Fraiberg, S. (1950). On the sleep disturbances of early childhood. *Psychoanalytic Study of the Child, 5,* 285-309.

Fraiberg, S. (1952). A critical neurosis in a two-and-a-half-year-old girl. *Psychoanalytic Study of the Child, 7,* 173-215.

Fraiberg, S. (1959). *The magic years: Understanding and handling the problems of early childhood.* New York: Scribner.

Fraiberg, S. (1977). *Insights from the blind.* New York: Basic Books.

Fraiberg, S. (1980). *Clinical studies in infant mental health: The first year of life.* New York: Basic Books.

Frankenburg, W. K., & Dodds, J. B. (1970). *The Denver developmental screening test.* Denver, CO: Ladoca Project.

Freud, A. (1945). Indications for child analysis. *Psychoanalytic Study of the Child, 1,* 131-149.

Freud, A. (1946). *The ego and the mechanisms of defence.* New York: International Universities Press.

Freud, A. (1954). Problems of infantile neurosis. *Psychoanalytic Study of the Child, 9,* 16-17.

Freud, A. (1962). Assessment of childhood disturbances. *Psychoanalytic Study of the Child, 17,* 149-158.

Freud, A. (1965). *Normality and pathology in childhood.* New York: International Universities Press.

Freud, A. (1968). Indications and contra-indications for child analysis. *Psychoanalytic Study of the Child, 23*, 37-46.

Freud, A., & Burlington, D. (1944). *Infants without families: The case for and against residential nurseries.* New York: International Universities Press.

Freud, S. (1953). *The interpretation of dreams* (1900). (Standard ed. vol. 4/5). London: Hogarth.

Freud, S. (1953). *Three essays on the theory of sexuality* (1905). (Standard ed. vol. 7). London: Hogarth.

Freud, S. (1955). *Analysis of a phobia of a five-year-old boy* (1909). (Standard ed. vol. 10). London: Hogarth.

Freud, S. (1955). *Beyond the pleasure principle* (1920). (Standard ed. vol. 18). London: Hogarth.

Freud, S. (1956). *An outline of psychoanalysis* (1940). (Standard ed. vol. 23). London: Hogarth.

Friedlander, K. (1946). Psychoanalytic orientation in child guidance work in Great Britain. *Psychoanalytic Study of the Child, 2*, 343-357.

Frommer, E. A., & O'Shea, G. (1973). Antenatal identification of women liable to have problems in managing their infants. *British Journal of Psychiatry, 123*, 149-156.

Fuchs, N. R. (1957). Play therapy at home. *Merrill-Palmer Quarterly, 3*, 89-95.

Gaensbauer, T. J., Mrazek, D., & Harmon, R. J. (1982). Behavioral observations of abused and/or neglected infants. In N. Frude (Ed.), *Psychological approaches to the understanding and prevention of child abuse.* London: Concord Books.

Gaensbauer, T. J., & Sands, K. (1979). Distorted affective communications in abused/neglected infants and their potential impact on caretakers. *Journal of the American Academy of Child Psychiatry, 18*, 236-250.

Galenson, E., & Roiphe, H. (1974). The emergence of genital awareness during the second year of life. In R. C. Friedman (Ed.), *Sex differences in behavior.* New York: Wiley.

Gardner, M. J. (1979). *Expressive one-word picture vocabulary test.* San Francisco: Academic Therapy Publication.

Garrison, F. H. (1965). History of pediatrics. In I. A. Abt (Ed.), *History of pediatrics* (Vol. 1). Philadelphia: Saunders.

Gerken, K. C. (1983). Assessment of preschool children with severe handicaps. In K. D. Paget & B. A. Bracken (Eds.), *The psychoeducational assessment of preschool children.* New York: Grune & Stratton.

Gesell, A. (1925). *The mental growth of the pre-school child.* New York: Macmillan.

Gesell, A. O., & Amatruda, C. S. (1964). *Developmental diagnosis* (11th ed.). New York: Harper & Row.

Ghodsian, M., Zajicek, E., & Wolkind, S. (1980). Maternal depression and child behaviour problems. *Journal of Child Psychology and Psychiatry, 25*, 91-109.

Goren, C. (1975, April). *Form perception, innate form preferences and visually-mediated head turning in human newborns.* Paper presented at the meeting of the Society for Research in Child Development, Denver.

Gottfried, A. W., & Gottfried, A. E. (1984). Home environment and cognitive development in young children of middle-socioeconomic-status families. In A. W. Gottfried (Ed.), *Home environment and early cognitive development: Longitudinal research.* Orlando, FL: Academic Press.

Greenspan, S. I. (1981). *Psychopathology and adaptation in infancy and early childhood.* New York: International Universities Press.

Griffiths, R. (1954). *The abilities of babies: A study in mental measurement.* New York: McGraw-Hill.

Guerney, B. (1964). Filial therapy. *Journal of Consulting Psychology, 28*, 304-310.

Guilhaume, A., Benoit, O., Gourmelen, M., & Richardet, J. M. (1982). Relationship between sleep stage IV deficit and reversible HGH deficiency in psychological dwarfism. *Pediatric Research, 16*, 299-303.

Gustafson, G., Green, J., & West, M. (1979). The infant's changing role in mother-infant games: The growth of social skills. *Infant Behavior and Development, 1*, 301-308.

Gutelins, M. F., Millican, F. K., Layman, E. M., Cohen, G. T., & Dublin, C. C. (1962). Nutritional studies in children with pica. *Pediatrics, 29*, 1012-1023.

Hall, C. S., & Lindzey, G. (1970). *Theories of personality* (2nd ed.). New York: Wiley.

Hannaway, P. (1976). Failure to thrive. A study of 100 infants and children. *Clinics in Pediatrics, 9*, 69-99.

Hardyment, C. (1984). *Dream babies*. New York: Oxford University Press.

Hartlage, O. C., & Telzrow, C. F. (1983). Neuropsychological assessment. In K. D. Paget & B. A. Bracken (Eds.), *The psychoeducational assessment of preschool children*. New York: Grune & Stratton.

Hartmann, H. (1958). *Ego psychology and the problem of adaptation*. New York: International Universities Press.

Henderson, J. L. (1953, August 8). The evolution of child care. *Lancet*, p. 261.

Hinde, R. A. (1982). *Ethology*. London: Fontana.

Hodapp, R. M., Goldfield, E. C., & Boyatzis, C. J. (1984). The use and effectiveness of maternal scaffolding in mother-infant games. *Child Development, 55*, 772-783.

Hoffer, P. C., & Hull, N.E.H. (1981). *Murdering mothers: Infanticide in England and New England 1558-1803*. New York: University Press.

Holt, L. E. (1897). *The diseases of infants and childhood for the use of students and practitioners of medicine*. New York: Appleton.

Holt, L. E. (1902). *The care and feeding of children*. New York: Appleton.

Hopkinson, K., Cox, A., & Rutter, M. (1981). Psychiatric interviewing techniques III. Naturalistic study: Eliciting feelings. *British Journal of Psychiatry, 138*, 406-415.

Hubert, N., Wachs, T. D., Peters, M. P. , & Gandour, M. (1982). The study of early temperament: Measurement and conceptual issues. *Child Development, 53*, 571-600.

Hunt, D. (1970). *Parents and children in history: The psychology of family life*. New York: Basic Books.

Illick, J. E. (1974). Child-rearing in seventeenth century England and America. In L. de Mause (Ed.), *The history of childhood*. New York: Psychohistory Press.

Illingworth, R. S., & Lister, J. (1964). The critical or sensitive period, with special reference to certain feeding problems in infants and children. *Journal of Pediatrics, 65*, 839-848.

Jacobs, L. (1949). Methods used in the education of mothers. *Psychoanalytic Study of the Child, 3/4*, 409-422.

Jenkins, S., Bax, M., & Hart, H. (1980). Behaviour problems in pre-school children. *Journal of Child Psychology and Psychiatry, 21*, 5-17.

Jenkins, S., Owen, C., Bax, M., & Hart, H. (1984). Continuities of common behaviour problems in preschool children. *Journal of Child Psychology and Psychiatry, 25*, 75-89.

Johnson, F. K., Dowling, J., & Wesner, D. (1980). Notes on infant psychotherapy. *Infant Mental Health Journal, 1*, 19-33.

Johnson, K. L., & Kopp, C. B. (1980). *A bibliography of screening and assessment measures for infants*. Unpublished manuscript, University of California, Los Angeles.

Jones, E., & Nisbett, R. (1971). *The actor and the observer: Divergent perceptions of the causes of behavior*. New York: General Learning Press.

Jones, M. C. (1924). The elimination of children's fears. *Journal of Experimental Psychology, 7*, 382-390.

Kagan, J. (1971). *Change and continuity in infancy.* New York: Wiley.

Kagan, J. (1981). *The second year.* Cambridge, MA: Harvard University Press.

Kagan, J. (1982). *Review of research in infancy.* New York: Grant Foundation Publication.

Kanner, L. (1944). Early infantile autism. *Journal of Pediatrics, 25,* 211-217.

Kessen, W. (1965). *The child.* New York: Wiley.

Kirk, S. A., McCarthy, J. J., & Kirk, W. D. (1968). *Illinois test of psycholinguistic abilities.* Urbana: University of Illinois Press.

Klaus, M. H., & Kennell, J. H. (1982). *Parent-infant bonding* (2nd ed.). St. Louis: Mosby.

Klein, M. (1960). *The psychoanalysis of children.* New York: Grove.

Kligman, D., Smyrl, R., & Emde, R. N. (1975). A "non-intrusive" home study of infant sleep. *Psychosomatic Medicine, 37,* 448-453.

Klinnert, M. D. (1984). Regulation of infant behavior by maternal facial expression. *Infant Behavior and Development, 7,* 447-465.

Klinnert, M. D., Campos, J., Sorce, J. F., Emde, R. N., et al. (1982). Social referencing: Emotional expressions as behavior regulators. In R. Plutchik & H. Kellerman (Eds.), *Emotions in early development.* New York: Academic Press.

Knobloch, H., & Pasamanick, B. (1974). *Gesell and Amatruda's developmental diagnosis.* Hagerstown, MD: Harper & Row.

Kopp, C. B. (1983). Risk factors in development. In P. H. Mussen (Ed.), *Handbook of child psychology: Vol. 2. Infancy and developmental psychobiology.* New York: Wiley.

Korner, A. F., & Thoman, E. B., (1972). Relative efficacy of contact and vestibular stimulation in soothing neonates. *Child Development, 43,* 443-453.

Krieger, I. (1982). *Pediatric disorders of feeding, nutrition, and metabolism.* New York: Wiley.

Langer, W. (1973/1974). Infanticide: A historical survey. *History of Childhood Quarterly, 1,* 354-365.

Lee, L. L. (1971). *The Northwestern syntax screening test.* Evanston, IL: Northwestern University Press.

Leonard, M. R. (1959). Fear of walking in a two-and-one-half-year-old girl. *Psychoanalytic Quarterly, 28,* 29-39.

Lewis, J. A. (1982). Oral motor assessment and treatment of feeding difficulties. In P. J. Accardo (Ed.), *Failure to thrive in infancy and childhood.* Baltimore: University Park Press.

Lewis, M., & Brooks-Gunn, J. (1979). *Social cognition and the acquisition of self.* New York: Plenum Press.

Lipsitt, L. P. (1983). Stress in infancy: Toward understanding the origins of coping behavior. In N. Garmezy & M. Rutter (Eds.), *Stress, coping and development in children.* New York: McGraw-Hill.

Lipton, E. L., Steinschneider, A., & Richmond, J. B. (1965). Swaddling, a child care practice: Historical, cultural and experimental observations. *Pediatrics, 35,* 520-567.

Locke, J. (1947). Some thoughts concerning education. In *John Locke on politics and education.* New York: Walter Black.

Lockyer, L., & Rutter, M. (1970). A five- to fifteen-year follow-up study of infantile psychosis: IV. Patterns of cognitive ability. *British Journal of Social and Clinical Psychology, 9,* 152-163.

Lorenz, K. (1950). Ganzheit und Teil in der tierischen und menschlichen Gemeinschaft. In *Ueber tierisches und menschliches Verhalten. Gesammelte Abhandlungen, Band I + II.* München: Piper.

Lovaas, I., Koegel, R., Simmons, J. Q., & Long, J. S. (1973). Some generalization and follow-up measures on autistic children in behavior therapy. *Journal of Applied Behavioral Analysis, 6*, 131-166.

Lozoff, B., Wolf, A. W., & Davis, N. S. (1985). Sleep problems in pediatric practice. *Pediatrics, 75*, 477-483.

Maccoby, E. E., & Jacklin, L. N. (1974). *The psychology of sex differences.* Stanford, CA: Stanford University Press.

Mahler, M. S. (1968). On human symbiosis and the vicissitudes of individuation. In *Infantile psychosis* (Vol. 1). New York: International Universities Press.

Mahler, M. S., & McDevitt, J. B. (1980). The separation-individuation process and identity formation. In S. I. Greenspan & C. H. Pollock (Eds.), *The course of life, I.* Bethesda, MD: National Institute of Mental Health.

Mahler, M. S., Pine, F., & Bergmann, A. (1975). *The psychological birth of the infant.* New York: Basic Books.

Mahrer, A. R., Levinson, J. R., & Fine, S. (1976). Infant psychotherapy: Theory, research, and practice. *Psychotherapy: Theory, Research and Practice, 13*, 131-140.

Main, M., & Weston, D. (1981). The quality of the toddler's relationship to mother and father: Related to conflict behavior and the readiness to establish new relationships. *Child Development, 52*, 932-940.

Marton, P., Minde, K., & Dawson, H. (1981). The role of the father for the infant at risk. *American Journal of Orthopsychiatry, 51*, 672-679.

Marvick, E. W. (1974). Nature versus nurture: Patterns and trends in seventeenth century French child-rearing. In L. de Mause (Ed.), *The history of childhood.* New York: Psychohistory Press.

Matas, L., Arend, R. A., & Sroufe, L. A. (1978). Continuity of adaptation in the second year of life: The relationship between quality of attachment and later competence. *Child Development, 49*, 547-556.

McAdoo, W., & deMyer, M. (1978). Personality characteristics of parents. In M. Rutter & E. Schopler (Eds.), *Autism: A reappraisal of concepts and treatment.* New York: Plenum Press.

McCall, R. B. (1979). The development of intellectual functioning in infancy and the prediction of later IQ. In J. D. Osofsky (Ed.), *Handbook of infant development.* New York: Wiley.

McCall, R. B. (1981). Nature-nurture and the two realms of development: A proposed integration with respect to mental development. *Child Development, 52*, 1-12.

McCarthy, D. (1972). *McCarthy Scales of Children's Abilities.* New York: Psychological Corporation.

McHale, S., Simeonsson, R., Marcus, L., & Olley, L. (1980). The social and symbolic quality of autistic children's communication. *Journal of Autism and Developmental Disorders, 10*, 299-310.

McLaughlin, M. M. (1974). Survivors and surrogates: Children and parents from the ninth to the thirteenth centuries. In L. de Mause (Ed.), *The history of childhood.* New York: Psychohistory Press.

Messick, S. (1983). Assessment of children. In P. H. Mussen (Ed.), *Handbook of child psychology: Vol. 1. History, theory and methods.* New York: Wiley.

Mikkelson, E. (1982). Efficacy of neuroleptic medication in pervasive developmental disorders of childhood. *Schizophrenia Bulletin, 8*, 320-332.

Minde, K. K. (1984). The impact of prematurity on the later behavior of children and on their families. *Clinics in Perinatology, 11*, 227-244.

Minde, K., Corter, C., & Goldberg, S. (1984). The contribution of twinship and health to early interaction and attachment between premature infants and their mothers. In

J. D. Call, E. Galenson, & R. L. Tyson (Eds.), *Frontiers of infant psychiatry II*. New York: Basic Books.

Minde, K., Marton, P., Manning, D., & Hines, B. (1980). Some determinants of mother-infant interaction in the premature nursery. *Journal of the American Academy of Child Psychiatry, 19*, 1-21.

Minde, K., & Minde, R. (1981). Psychiatric intervention in infancy: A review. *Journal of the American Academy of Child Psychiatry, 20*, 217-238.

Minde, K., & Perotta, M. (1985). Maternal perception and mother-infant interaction in developmentally delayed premature infants. Manuscript submitted for publication.

Minde, K., Shosenberg, N., Marton, P., Thompson, J., Ripley, J., & Burns, S. (1980). Self-help groups in a premature nursery: A controlled evaluation. *Journal of Pediatrics, 96*, 933-940.

Minde, K., Webb, G., & Sykes, D. (1968). Studies on the hyperactive child VI: Prenatal and paranatal factors associated with hyperactivity. *Developmental Medicine and Child Neurology, 10*, 355-367.

Moore, T., & Ucko, L. (1957). Night waking in early infancy: Part 1. *Archives of Disease in Childhood, 32*, 333-342.

Moss, H. (1967). Sex, age and state as determinants of mother-infant interaction. *Merrill-Palmer Quarterly, 13*, 19-36.

Mrazek, D. A. (1984). Effects of hospitalization on early child development. In R. N. Emde & R. J. Harmon (Eds.), *Continuities and discontinuities in development*. New York: Plenum Press.

Neubauer, P. B. (1972). Psychoanalysis of the preschool child. In B. Wolman (Ed.), *Handbook of child psychoanalysis*. New York: Van Nostrand.

Newson, J., & Newson, E. (1976). *Seven years old in the home environment*. London: Allen & Unwin.

Nicolich, L. M. (1977). Beyond sensorimotor intelligence: Assessment of symbolic maturity through analysis of pretend play. *Merrill-Palmer Quarterly, 23*, 89-99.

Ornitz, E. M., Guthrie, D., & Farley, A. H. (1977). The early development of autistic children. *Journal of Autism and Childhood Schizophrenia, 7*, 207-229.

Ottinger, D. R., & Simmons, J. E. (1964). Behavior of human neonates and prenatal maternal anxiety. *Psychological Reports, 14*, 391-394.

Palmer, S., Thompson, R. J., & Linscheid, T. R. (1975). Applied behavior analysis in the treatment of childhood feeding problems. *Developmental Medicine and Child Neurology, 17*, 333-339.

Papousek, H., & Papousek, M. (1979). Early ontogeny of human social interaction. In M. von Cranach, K. Foppa, W. Lepenies, & D. Ploog (Eds.), *Human ethology*. Cambridge: Cambridge University Press.

Parmelee, A. H. (1974). Ontogeny of sleep patterns and associated periodicities in infants. In S. R. Berenberg, M. Caniaris, & N. P. Masse (Eds.), *Pre- and postnatal development of the human brain* (Vol. 13). Basel: S. Karger.

Parmelee, A. H., Wenner, W. H., & Schulz, H. R. (1964). Infant sleep patterns; From birth to 16 weeks of age. *Journal of Pediatrics, 65*, 576-582.

Peiper, A. (1966). *Quellen zur Kinderheilkunde*. Bern: Huber.

Pestalozzi, J. H. (1900). *How Gertrude teaches her children* (L. Holland & F. Turner, Trans.). London: Swann-Sonnenschein. (Original work published 1801)

Piaget, J. (1952). *The origin of intelligence in children*. New York: International Universities Press.

Piaget, J. (1969). The intellectual development of the adolescent. In G. Caplan & S. Lebovici (Eds.), *Adolescence: Psycho-social perspectives*. New York: Basic Books.

Pliny the Elder (1942). *Natural history* (Book VII). H. Rackham. Cambridge, MA: Harvard University Press.

Pollitt, E. (1975). Failure to thrive: Socioeconomic, dietary intake, and mother-child interaction data. *Federal Proceedings, 34,* 1593-1597.

Pollock, L. A. (1983). *Forgotten children: Parent-child relations from 1500 to 1900.* Cambridge: Cambridge University Press.

Potter, H. W. (1933). Schizophrenia in children. *American Journal of Psychiatry, 89,* 1253-1270.

Prechtl, H.F.R. (1974). The behavioural states of the newborn infant (a review). *Brain Research, 76,* 1404-1411.

Prechtl, H.F.R. (1982). Assessment methods for the newborn infant: A critical evaluation. In T. Stratton (Ed.), *Psychobiology of the human newborn.* Chichester: Wiley.

Prechtl, H.F.R. (1985, January). *A new look at early development of the fetus and young infant.* Paper presented at the International Symposium on Psychobiology and Early Development, Berlin.

Prechtl, H.F.R., Akiyama, Y., Zinkin, P., & Kerr Grant, D. (1968). Polygraphic studies of the full term newborn. II. Computer analysis of recorded data. In M. Bax & R. MacKeith (Eds.), *Clinics in developmental medicine* (Vol. 27). London: Heinemann.

Prechtl, H.F.R., & Beintema, D. (1964). The neurological examination of the full term newborn infant. *Little Club Clinics in Developmental Medicine, No. 12.* London: Spastics Society.

Provence, S. (1972). Psychoanalysis and the treatment of psychological disorders of infancy. In B. B. Wolman (Ed.), *Handbook of child psychoanalysis.* New York: Van Nostrand Reinhold.

Provence, S. (1974). Some relationships between activity and vulnerability in the early years. In J. Anthony & C. Chiland (Eds.), *The child in his family* (vol. 3). New York: Wiley.

Provence, S. (1978). Application of psychoanalytic principles to treatment and prevention in infancy. In J. Glenn (Ed.), *Child analysis and therapy.* New York: Aronson.

Provence, S., Leonard, M., & Naylor, A. (1982). *Developmental diagnosis: An approach to assessing mental health in infants.* Presented at Congress of the International Association for Child and Adolescent Psychiatry and Allied Professions, Dublin, Ireland.

Provence, S., & Lipton, R. (1962). *Infants in institutions.* New York: International Universities Press.

Provence, S., & Naylor, A. (1983). *Working with disadvantaged parents and their children.* New Haven, CT: Yale University Press.

Prugh, D. G., & Eckhardt, L. O. (1980). Children's reactions to illness, hospitalization, and surgery. In H. I. Kaplan, A. M. Freedman, & B. J. Sadock (Eds.), *Comprehensive textbook of psychiatry* (Vol. 3). Baltimore: Williams & Wilkins.

Prugh, D. G., Straub, E. M., Sands, H. H., Kirschbaum, R. M., & Lenihan, E. A. (1953). A study of the emotional reactions of children and families to hospitalization and illness. *American Journal of Orthopsychiatry, 23,* 70-106.

Quinton, D., & Rutter, M. (1976). Early hospital admissions and later disturbances of behavior: An attempted replication of Douglas' findings. *Developmental Medicine and Child Neurology, 18,* 447-459.

Ramey, C. T., Bryant, D. M., Sparling, J. J., & Wasik, B. H. (1984). *A biosocial systems perspective on environmental interventions for low birthweight infants.* Manuscript in preparation.

Ramey, C. T., MacPhee, D., & Yeates, K. O. (1982). Preventing developmental retardation. A general systems model. In L. Bond & J. Joffe (Eds.), *Facilitating infant and early childhood development.* Hanover, NH: University Press of New England.

Ramey, C. T., & Trohanis, P. L. (Eds.). (1982). *Finding and educating high-risk and handicapped infants.* Baltimore: University Park Press.

Rapaport, D. (1951). Toward a theory of thinking. In *Organization and pathology of thought*. New York: Columbia University Press.

Rapaport, D. (1959). A historical survey of psychoanalytic ego psychology. *Psychological Issues, 1*, 5-17.

Ray-Grant, Q., Carr, R., & Berman, G. (1983). Childhood developmental disorders. In P. D. Steinhauer & Q. Ray-Grant (Eds.), *Psychological problems of the child in the family*. New York: Basic Books.

Reynell, J. (1977). *Reynell developmental language scales (RDLS). Manual (Revised Ed.)*. Windsor, England: NFER.

Reynell, J., & Zinkin, P. (1975). New procedures for the developmental assessment of young children with severe visual handicaps. *Child Care, Health and Development, 61*, 61-69.

Richman, N. (1981). A community survey of characteristics of one- to two-year-olds with sleep disturbances. *Journal of the American Academy of Child Psychiatry, 20*, 281-291.

Richman, N. (1985). A double blind drug trial of treatment in young children with waking problems. *Journal of Child Psychology and Psychiatry, 20*, 281-291.

Richman, N., Douglas, J., Hunt, H., Lansdown, R., & Levere, R. (1985). Behavioural methods in the treatment of sleep disorders—a pilot study. *Journal of Child Psychology and Psychiatry, 20*, 581-590.

Richman, N., Stevenson, J., & Graham, P. J. (1982). *Pre-school to school: A behavioural study*. London: Academic Press.

Ritvo, E. R. (1977). Biochemical studies of children with the syndromes of autism, childhood schizophrenia and related developmental disabilities: A review. *Journal of Child Psychology and Psychiatry, 18*, 373-379.

Ritvo, E. R., Ornitz, E. M., Walter, R. D., & Hanley, J. (1970). Correlation of psychiatric diagnoses and EEG findings: A double-blind study of 184 hospitalized children. *American Journal of Psychiatry, 126*, 988-996.

Robertson, J. (1953). Some responses of young children to loss of maternal care. *Nursing Times, 49*, 382-386.

Robertson, J., & Bowlby, J. (1952). Responses of young children to separation from their mothers. *Courrier: Centre internationale de l'enfante, 2*, 131-142.

Robertson, P. (1974). Home as a nest: Middle class childhood in nineteenth-century Europe. In L. de Mause (Ed.), *The history of childhood*. New York: Psychohistory Press.

Roffwarg, H. P., Clark, R. W., Guilleminault, C., Hauri, P. J., Kupfer, D. J., Miles, L. E., Schmidt, H. S., Zarcone, V. P., & Zorick, F. J. (1979). Diagnostic classification of sleep and arousal disorders. Sleep Disorders Classification Committee, Association of Sleep Disorders Centers. *Sleep, 2*, 21-121.

Roiphe, H., & Galenson, E. (1981). *Infantile origin of sexual identity*. New York: International Universities Press.

Rosenblith, J. F. (1974). Relations between neonatal behaviors and those at eight months. *Developmental Psychology, 10*, 779-792.

Ross, J. B., & McLaughlin, M. M. (1949). *The portable medieval reader*. New York: Viking Press.

Rousseau, J. J. (1979). *Emile* (Allan Bloom, Trans.). New York: Basic Books. (Originally published 1762).

Rutter, M. (1970). Autistic children: Infancy to adulthood. *Seminars in Psychiatry, 2*, 435-450.

Rutter, M. (1970). Psychological development: Predictions from infancy. *Journal of Child Psychology and Psychiatry, 11*, 49-62.

Rutter, M. (1981). *Maternal deprivation reassessed* (2nd ed.). Harmondsworth, Middlesex: Penguin.

Rutter, M. (1983). Cognitive deficits in the pathogenesis of autism. *Journal of Child Psychology and Psychiatry. 24,* 513-531.

Rutter, M. (1984). Continuities and discontinuities in socioemotional development. In R. N. Emde & R. J. Harmon (Eds.), *Continuities and discontinuities in development.* New York: Plenum Press.

Rutter, M., Greenfield, D., & Lockyer, L. (1967). A five to fifteen year follow-up study of infantile psychosis: II: Social and behavioral outcome. *British Journal of Psychiatry, 113,* 1183-1199.

Rutter, M., Yule, B., Quinton, D., Rowlands, O., Yule, W., & Berger, M. (1975). Attainment and adjustment in two geographical areas—Some factors accounting for area differences. *British Journal of Psychiatry, 126,* 520-533.

Sainte Marthe, S. (1797). *Paedotrophia, A didactic poem.* (H. Tytler, Trans.). London: Nichols.

Sameroff, A. J., & Chandler, M. J. (1975). Reproductive risk and the continuum of caretaking casualty. In F. D. Horowitz, M. Hetherington, S. Scarr-Salapatek, & G. Siegal (Eds.), *Review of child development research* (Vol. 4). Chicago: University of Chicago Press.

Sander, L. (1970). Early mother-infant interaction and twenty-four hour patterns of activity and sleep. *Journal of the American Academy of Child Psychiatry, 9,* 103-123.

Sander, L. (1975). Infant and caretaking environment: Investigation and conceptualization of adaptive behavior in a system of increasing complexity. In E. J. Anthony (Ed.), *Explorations in child psychiatry.* New York: Plenum Press.

Sander, L. (1980). Investigation of the infant and its caregiving environment as a biological system. In S. I. Greenspan & G. H. Pollock (Eds.), *The course of life: Psychoanalytic contributions toward understanding personality development: Vol. 1. Infancy and early childhood.* Washington, DC: National Institute of Mental Health.

Sattler, J. M. (1974). *Assessment of children's intelligence.* Philadelphia: Saunders.

Schaefer, C. E., & Millman, H. L. (Eds.). (1977). *Therapies for children: A handbook of effective treatments for problem children.* San Francisco: Jossey-Bass.

Schaefer, E. S. (1981). Development of adaptive behavior: Conceptual models and family correlates. In M. Begab, H. Garber, & H. C. Haywood (Eds.), *Prevention of retarded development in psychosocially disadvantaged children.* Baltimore: University Park Press.

Schopler, E., Andrews, C. E., & Strupp, K. (1979). Do autistic children come from upper-middle class parents? *Journal of Autism and Developmental Disorders, 9,* 139-146.

Schulman, A. H., & Kaplowitz, C. (1977). Mirror-image response during the first two years of life. *Developmental Psychobiology, 10,* 133-142.

Schwartz, H. (1950). The mother in the consulting room. *Psychoanalytic Study of the Child, 5,* 349-357.

Sears, S. R., Maccoby, E. E., & Levin, H. (1957). *Patterns of child rearing.* New York: Row, Peterson.

Self, P. A., & Horowitz, F. D. (1979). The behavioral assessment of the neonate: An overview. In J. D. Osovsky (Ed.), *Handbook of infant development.* New York: Wiley.

Shapiro, V., Fraiberg, S., & Adelson, E. (1976). Infant-parent psychotherapy on behalf of a child in a critical nutritional state. *Psychoanalytic Study of the Child, 31,* 461-491.

Sigman, M., & Ungerer, J. (in press). Attachment behaviors in autistic and normal children. *Journal of Autism and Developmental Disorders.*

Sigman, M., Ungerer, J., Mundy, P., & Sherman, T. (1985). Cognitive functioning in autistic children. In D. Cohen, A. Donnellan, & R. Paul (Eds.), *Handbook of autism and disorders of atypical development.* New York: Wiley.

Silver, H. D., & Finkelstein, M. (1967). Deprivation dwarfism. *Journal of Pediatrics, 70,* 317-324.

Skinner, B. F. (1953). *Science and human behavior.* New York: Macmillan.

Smith, M. W. (1974). Alfred Binet's remarkable questions: A cross-national and cross-temporal analysis of the cultural biases built into the Stanford-Binet intelligence scale and other Binet tests. *Genetic Psychology Monographs, 89,* 307-334.

Sorce, J. F., & Emde, R. N. (1981). Mother's presence is not enough. *Developmental Psychology, 17,* 737-745.

Sparrow, S. S., Balla, D. A., & Cicchetti, D. V. (1984). *Vineland adaptive behavior scales: A revision of the Vineland social maturity scale by Edgar A. Doll.* Circle Pines, MN: American Guidance Service.

Sperling, M. (1952). Animal phobia in a 2-year-old child. *Psychoanalytic Study of the Child, 7,* 117-125.

Spitz, R. (1945). Hospitalism: An inquiry into the genesis of psychiatric conditions in early childhood. *Psychoanalytic Study of the Child, 1,* 53-74.

Spitz, R. (1946). Hospitalism: A follow-up report. *Psychoanalytic Study of the Child, 2,* 113-117.

Spitz, R. (1961). Some early prototypes of ego defences. *Journal of the American Psychoanalytic Association, 9,* 626-651.

Spitz, R. (1965). *The first year of life: A psychoanalytic study of normal and deviant development of object relations.* New York: International Universities Press.

Spitz, R., & Wolf, K. (1946). Anaclitic depression: An inquiry into the genesis of psychiatric conditions in early childhood. *Psychoanalytic Study of the Child, 2,* 313-342.

Spock, B. (1946). *The common sense book of baby and child care.* New York: Duell, Sloan.

Sroufe, L. A. (1979). Socioemotional development. In J. D. Osofsky (Ed.), *Handbook of infant development.* New York: Wiley.

Sroufe, L. A., Waters, E., & Matas, L. (1974). Contextual determinants of infant affective response. In M. Lewis & L. Rosenblum (Eds.), *The origins of fear.* New York: Wiley.

Steinhauer, P. D., & Rae-Grant, Q. (1983). *Psychological problems of the child in the family.* New York: Basic Books.

Sterba, E. (1941). An important factor in eating disturbances in childhood. *Psychoanalytic Quarterly, 10,* 365-372.

Sterba, E. (1949). Analysis of psychogenic constipation in a two-year-old child. *Psychoanalytic Study of the Child, 3/4,* 227-252.

Stern, D. (1974). Mother and infant at play: The dyadic interaction involving facial, vocal and gaze behaviors. In M. Lewis & L. Rosenblum (Eds.), *The effect of the infant on its caregiver.* New York: Wiley.

Stern, D. N. (1984). Affect attunement. In J. D. Call, E. Galenson, & R. L. Tyson (Eds.), *Frontiers of infant psychiatry II.* New York: Basic Books.

Stern, D. N., Barnett, R. K., & Spieker, S. (1982). Early transmission of affect: Some research issues. In J. D. Call, E. Galenson, & R. L. Tyson (Eds.), *Frontiers of infant psychiatry I.* New York: Basic Books.

Still, G. F. (1931). *The history of paediatrics.* Oxford: Oxford University Press.

Thomas, A. (1981). Current trends in developmental theory. *American Journal of Orthopsychiatry, 51,* 580-609.

Thomas, A., Chess, S., & Birch, H. G. (1968). *Temperament and behavior disorders in children.* New York: New York University Press.

Thomas, A., Chess, S., Birch, H. G., Herzog, M., & Kern, S. (1963). *Behavioral individuality in early childhood*. New York: New York University Press.

Thompson, M., & Havelkova, M. (1983). Psychoses in childhood and adolescence. In P. D. Steinhauer & Q. Rae-Grant (Eds.), *Psychological problems of the child in the family*. New York: Basic Books.

Tinbergen, E. A., & Tinbergen, N. (1976). The aetiology of childhood autism: A criticism of the Tinbergen's theory: A rejoinder. *Psychological Medicine, 6*, 545-550.

Trexler, R. C. (1973). Infanticide in Florence: New sources and first results. *History of Childhood Quarterly, 1*, 98-116.

Tronick, E., Ricks, M., & Cohn, J. (1982). Maternal and infant affective exchange: Patterns of adaptation. In T. Field & A. Fogel (Eds.), *Emotion and early interaction*. Hillsdale, NJ: Erlbaum.

Uzgiris, I. C., & Hunt, J. McV. (1975). *Ordinal scales of psychological development*. Urbana: University of Illinois Press.

Volkmar, R. R., & Cohen, D. J. (1985). Pervasive developmental disorders. In *Psychiatry*. Cavenar, NJ: Lippincott.

Wachs, T. D. (1978). The relationship of infants' physical environment to their Binet performance at 2½ years. *International Journal of Behavioral Development, 1*, 51-65.

Wachs, T. D. (1979). Proximal experience and early cognitive-intellectual development: The physical environment. *Merrill-Palmer Quarterly, 25*, 3-41.

Ward, A. J. (1970). Early infantile autism: Diagnosis, etiology and treatment. *Psychological Bulletin, 73*, 350-362.

Waters, E., Wippmann, J., & Sroufe, L. A. (1979). Attachment, positive affect, and competence in the peer group: Two studies in construct validation. *Child Development, 50*, 821-829.

Watson, J. B. (1924). *Behaviorism*. New York: Norton.

Watson, J. B. (1928). *Psychological care of infant and child*. New York: Norton.

Watson, J. B., & Rayner, R. (1920). Conditioned emotional reactions. *Journal of Experimental Psychology, 3*, 1-14.

Werner, E. E. (1972). Denver developmental screening test. In O. K. Buros (Ed.), *Seventh mental measurement yearbook* (Vol. 1). Highland Park, NJ: Gryphon Press.

Werner, H. (1948). *Comparative psychology of mental development* (rev. ed.). Chicago: Follett.

White, R. W. (1959). Motivation reconsidered: The concept of competence. *Psychological Review, 66*, 297-333.

Williams, C. D. (1959). The elimination of tantrum behavior by extinction procedures. *Journal of Abnormal Social Psychology, 59*, 269-277.

Wilson, R. S. (1977). Mental development in twins. In A. Oliverio (Ed.), *Genetics, environment and intelligence*. Amsterdam: North-Holland.

Wing, L. (1981). Sex ratios in early childhood autism and related conditions. *Psychiatric Research, 5*, 129-139.

Wing, L., & Gould, J. (1979). Severe impairments of social interaction and associated abnormalities in children: Epidemiology and classification. *Journal of Autism and Developmental Disorders, 9*, 11-29.

Winnicott, D. (1960). The theory of the parent-infant relationship. *International Journal of Psychoanalysis, 41*, 585-595.

Wolff, P. H. (1966). The causes, controls and organization of behavior in the neonate. *Psychological Issues, 5* (whole No. 17).

Wolff, P. H. (1969). Crying and vocalization in early infancy. In B. Foss (Ed.), *Determinants of infant behavior IV*. New York: Wiley.

Wolkind, S. N. (1977). Women who have been "in care"—psychological and social status during pregnancy. *Journal of Child Psychology and Psychiatry, 18*, 179-182.

Woolston, J. L. (1983). Eating disorders in infancy and early childhood. *Journal of the American Academy of Child Psychiatry, 22*, 114-121.

Yang, R. K. (1979). Early infant assessment: An overview. In J. D. Osovsky (Ed.), *Handbook of infant development*. New York: Wiley.

Yarrow, L. H., Morgan, G. A., Jennings, K. D., Harmon, R. J., & Gaiter, J. L. (1982). Infants' persistence at tasks: Relationships to cognitive functioning and early experience. *Infant Behavior and Development, 5*, 131-141.

Yarrow, L. J., & Pederson, F. A. (1976). The interplay between cognition and motivation in infants. In M. Lewis (Ed.), *Origins of intelligence*. New York: Plenum Press.

Yarrow, L. J., Rubenstein, J., & Pedersen, F. (1975). *Infant and environment*. New York: Wiley.

Young, G. J., Kavanagh, M. E., Anderson, G. M., Shaywitz, B. A., & Cohen, D. J. (1982). Clinical neurochemistry of autism and associated disorders. *Journal of Autism and Developmental Disorders, 12*, 147-157.

Zelazo, P. R. (1982). Alternative assessment procedures for handicapped infants and toddlers. In D. D. Bricker (Ed.), *Intervention with at-risk and handicapped infants*. Baltimore: University Park Press.

Zimmerman, I. L., Steiner, V. G., & Ewatt, R. L. (1969). *Preschool language scale*. Columbus, OH: Merrill.

INDEX

ABOUT THE AUTHORS

Klaus Minde, M.D., is currently Professor of Psychiatry and Pediatrics at the University of Toronto. He is an authority on infant psychiatry, although his research over the last two decades has spanned several central areas within the field of child psychiatry including family studies, hyperactivity, and psychopharmacology. Much of his work has addressed important issues in the interface of pediatrics and child psychiatry.

Regina Minde has a Ph.D. in Slavic Studies but has since obtained additional training in psychology. She is actively involved in collaborative research and writing projects with Klaus Minde.